Cancer Etiology, Diagnosis and Treatments

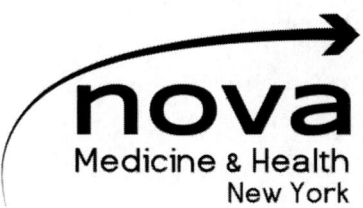

Cancer Etiology, Diagnosis and Treatments

Precision Cancer Immunotherapy
Andrey S. Bryukhovetskiy, MD, PhD,
Hari Shanker Sharma and Aruna Sharma
2023. ISBN: 979-8-88697-624-3 (eBook)

**Platinum-Based Chemotherapy:
Clinical Uses, Efficacy and Side Effects**
Kulmira Nurgali, PhD
and Raquel Abalo Delgado, PhD (Editors)
2022. ISBN: 978-1-68507-972-7 (Hardcover)
2022. ISBN: 979-8-88697-262-7 (eBook)

How Plant Flavonoids Affect the Outcome of Hormonal and Biological Cancer Therapies: A Handbook for Doctors and Patients
Katrin Sak, PhD
2022. ISBN: 978-1-68507-608-5 (Hardcover)
2022. ISBN: 978-1-68507-698-6 (eBook)

Burkitt Lymphoma: Diagnosis, Risk Factors and Treatment
Douglas V. Berthelot (Editor)
2021. ISBN: 978-1-68507-071-7 (Hardcover)
2021. ISBN: 978-1-68507-083-0 (eBook)

Bridging the Gap: In This Era of Cancer Immunotherapy
Shiu Y. Tsao, FRCR (Editor)
2021. ISBN: 978-1-53619-900-0 (Hardcover)
2021. ISBN: 978-1-53619-983-3 (eBook)

More information about this series can be found at
https://novapublishers.com/product-category/series/cancer-etiology-diagnosis-and-treatments/

Joseph Gerfried
Editor

New Research on Bone Metastasis

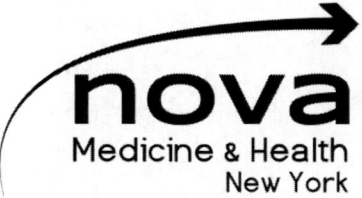

Copyright © 2023 by Nova Science Publishers, Inc.

All rights reserved. No part of this book may be reproduced, stored in a retrieval system or transmitted in any form or by any means: electronic, electrostatic, magnetic, tape, mechanical photocopying, recording or otherwise without the written permission of the Publisher.

We have partnered with Copyright Clearance Center to make it easy for you to obtain permissions to reuse content from this publication. Please visit copyright.com and search by Title, ISBN, or ISSN.

For further questions about using the service on copyright.com, please contact:

Copyright Clearance Center
Phone: +1-(978) 750-8400 Fax: +1-(978) 750-4470 E-mail: info@copyright.com

NOTICE TO THE READER

The Publisher has taken reasonable care in the preparation of this book but makes no expressed or implied warranty of any kind and assumes no responsibility for any errors or omissions. No liability is assumed for incidental or consequential damages in connection with or arising out of information contained in this book. The Publisher shall not be liable for any special, consequential, or exemplary damages resulting, in whole or in part, from the readers' use of, or reliance upon, this material. Any parts of this book based on government reports are so indicated and copyright is claimed for those parts to the extent applicable to compilations of such works.

Independent verification should be sought for any data, advice or recommendations contained in this book. In addition, no responsibility is assumed by the Publisher for any injury and/or damage to persons or property arising from any methods, products, instructions, ideas or otherwise contained in this publication.

This publication is designed to provide accurate and authoritative information with regards to the subject matter covered herein. It is sold with the clear understanding that the Publisher is not engaged in rendering legal or any other professional services. If legal or any other expert assistance is required, the services of a competent person should be sought. FROM A DECLARATION OF PARTICIPANTS JOINTLY ADOPTED BY A COMMITTEE OF THE AMERICAN BAR ASSOCIATION AND A COMMITTEE OF PUBLISHERS.

Library of Congress Cataloging-in-Publication Data

ISBN: 979-8-88697-799-8

Published by Nova Science Publishers, Inc. † New York

Contents

Preface vii

Chapter 1   **The Crucial Role of m⁶A Modification in Bone Cancer Metastases** 1
Chuan Yang, Zihan Deng and Yueqi Chen

Chapter 2   **The "Communicator" Role of Extracellular Vesicles in Bone Metastasis** 27
Zicai Dong and Yueqi Chen

Chapter 3   **Metastatic Disease of the Spine** 41
Balaji Zacharia

Chapter 4   **The Crucial Role of Estrogen and Relevant Receptors in Cancer Associated Bone Metastasis** 71
Yiran Wang

Chapter 5   **Evolving Cancer–Bone Coupling Effects During Bone Metastasis** 85
Fangze Xing, Hui Qiang and Pei Yang

Chapter 6   **Macrophages' Promotion of Bone Metastasis** 99
Zhiguo Ling and Yueqi Chen

Index 113

Preface

This book focuses on the latest developments in bone metastasis research, including:

- The application of m6A in the early diagnosis and therapeutic implications of bone metastasis
- The role of extracellular vesicles in bone metastasis
- The role of estrogen in affecting the immunological microenvironment of bone metastasis
- The etiology, pathogenesis, presentations, investigations, classification and management of spinal metastasis
- The pivotal role macrophages play in bone metastasis
- The evolving cancer-bone coupling effects during bone metastasis.

Chapter 1 - Bone is the most common site for metastasis in solid tumors, especially breast and prostate cancer. Bone metastasis, which causes a range of complications including bone pain, hypercalcemia, and fragility fracture, is a formidable challenge in cancer treatment and a leading cause of cancer mortality. N(6)-methyladenosine (m6A) is the most widespread and conserved posttranscriptional modification in cellular RNAs that regulates nearly all metabolism processes of RNAs, including RNA splicing, stability, nuclear export, and translation. Emerging evidence suggests that m6A is widely involved in cancer progression, such as tumorigenesis, proliferation, and metastasis. Although the specific mechanisms underlying bone metastasis remain unclear, increasing studies prove that m6A performs dual roles in bone metastasis *in situ* of osteosarcoma (OS) and distant bone metastasis of prostate cancer (PCa) and breast cancer (BCa).

In the present chapter, the authors summarized recent research on m6A modification and aimed to establish a theoretical basis for the application of m6A in the early diagnosis and therapeutic implications of bone metastasis.

Chapter 2 - Cancer-associated bone metastasis acts as the critical poor progression for the malignant tumors, which may be involved in the procedure of bone remodeling including osteoclasts-mediated bone resorption and osteoblasts-mediated bone regeneration. Several crucial cytokines secreted among osteoclasts and osteoblasts could make close interaction to promote cell differentiation, maturation and perform functions. In addition, many cell factors such as transforming growth factor beta (TGF-β), fibroblast growth factor (FGF), insulin growth factor (IGF), platelet-derived growth factor (PDGF), and bone morphogenetic proteins (BMPs) from the bone matrix during bone resorption lesions could induce the differentiation of MSCs into osteoblasts. In turn, osteoblasts might participate in osteoclastogenesis through secreting M-CSF and RANKL. Tumor associated bone metastasis exhibits osteolytic and osteogenic lesions. Extracellular vesicles could make coupling effects on bone remodeling process through their complex vesicular contents such as non-coding RNA, protein and so on.

In this chapter, the authors have summarized the role of extracellular vesicles in the procedure of bone metastasis during the micro-environment. In detail, it is well illustrated how breast cancer cell-derived extracellular vesicles affect the proliferation, differentiation and functions of osteoblasts and osteoclasts. In addition, it is also noted that the extracellular vesicles modulate the distant metastasis procedure of multiple myeloma and osteosarcoma from the original site to bone tissue. Elaborating on the role of extracellular vesicles in tumor associated bone metastasis may provide novel insight for the treatment of tumor bone metastasis.

Chapter 3 - The spine is the most common site of skeletal metastasis. The breast, prostate, lung, thyroid, and kidney are the tumors metastasizing to the spine. Hematogenous spread through the Batson plexus is the most typical mode of spread. Back pain is a common symptom. Spine metastasis also leads to vertebral compression fractures, deformity, and neurological deficits. Radiologically, there are osteolytic, osteosclerotic, and mixed types. Some metastases are radiosensitive, and others are radioresistant. Routine blood investigations, serum calcium, phosphorus, alkaline phosphatase, radiographs of the spine and chest, contrast-enhanced CT scan of the abdomen and chest, bone scans, and PET scans are common investigations. Primary tumor, epidural compression, type of lesion, stability of the segment, and general health of the patient influence the treatment. Treatment is a multimodal approach. Radiotherapy, stereotactic surgery, surgery combined with radiotherapy, and decompressive surgery are various modalities of treatment.

In this chapter, the authors describe the etiology, pathogenesis, presentations, investigations, classifications, and management of spinal metastasis.

Chapter 4 - Cancer associated metastasis is a unique and special characteristic of malignant tumors during poor progression. Even bone acts as the common tissue to become colonization site due to the tendency of solid tumors, including breast cancer (BCa) and prostate cancer (PCa). Then the osteolytic and osteogenic lesions could be performed during the procedure of bone metastasis. Additionally, bone matrix erosion and regeneration were closely associated with the metabolism of estrogen. In recent years, it has been illustrated that estrogen can play the critical role in affecting the immunological microenvironment of the bone metastasis.

In this chapter, the authors summarize the impacts of estrogen on immune cells and their consequences on bone homeostasis, metastasis settlement into the bone and relevant poor progression. In addition, the promising application of cancer associated bone metastasis is also discussed by targeting estrogen and its associated receptors.

Chapter 5 - Uncontrolled development, invasion, and metastasis are characteristics of cancer, the leading cause of death among patients worldwide. After the lung and liver, the bone marrow is the third most typical location for tumor spread. Tumor cells can escape with the primary tumor site, be customized to the bone microenvironment, and use the bone as a launch pad for further metastasis to other organs. As the tumor cells travel from the primary focus to the bone, they establish interactions with the bone microenvironment, and these interactions determine the fate of the cancer cells.

Bone is a highly dynamic tissue whose dynamic balance is coordinated by osteoclasts that destroy bone, osteoblasts that form bone, and mechanosensory osteoclasts. The interaction of hormones, paracrine growth factors, and cytokines also regulates this dynamic process. As a person ages, catabolism predominates in bone metabolism, and year-on-year bone loss reduces the strength of the bone while weakening its ability to repair damage caused by malignant infiltrative disease. The bone marrow can act as a remote responder for tumors at the primary focus and as a source of cells that recruit other organs to form premetastatic niche formation. Most tumor cells that leave the primary site are destroyed before they can establish metastasis. However, a small proportion of the surviving tumor cells are attracted by chemotaxis to the 'metastatic niche' in the hematopoietic bone marrow.

The first niche of disseminated tumor cells (DTC) in the bone microenvironment plays an essential role in subsequent metastasis. Tumor cells can induce osteoblasts to secrete RANKL by secreting osteolytic factors, which regulate osteoclastogenesis. Resorption of the bone matrix by over-activated osteoclasts leads to the release of numerous cytokines, which further act on the cancer cells to form an osteolytic vicious cycle. This process causes events such as bone marrow compression and pathological fractures. The asymptomatic phase of bone colonization may last for several years and is characterized by resting disseminated tumor cells with proliferating bone micrometastases, based on which the elimination of the tumourigenic capacity of DTC and BMM can effectively eliminate dormant cancer cells. The metastasis-limiting interactions of tumor cells with various cellular and non-cellular components of the bone marrow niche provide precious therapeutic targets.

Chapter 6 - Bone metastasis is a major cause of cancer-related mortality and treatment failure. Current strategies for treating bone metastasis are primarily aimed at relieving symptoms and slowing the progression of the disease, which fails to produce effective therapeutic outcomes. Therefore, it is critical to develop highly effective and promising therapeutic strategies.

Macrophages are the primary component of the tumor microenvironment and are key to tumor growth, invasion, and distant metastasis. Disruption of bone homeostasis is often a result of bone metastasis and thus restoring bone homeostasis is essential for successful treatment. Targeting macrophages may be a potential therapeutic option for restoring bone homeostasis due to their role as regulators. In addition, compelling clinical and scientific evidence has shown that macrophages could facilitate the multi-step progression of bone metastasis. Intriguingly, macrophages interact not only with cancer cells but also with local stromal cells, such as osteoclasts and osteoblasts, within the bone microenvironment, resulting in further bone metastasis deterioration.

In this chapter, the authors provide an overview of the pivotal role macrophages play in bone metastasis, as well as discuss promising strategies for targeting macrophages for bone metastasis treatment.

Chapter 1

The Crucial Role of m⁶A Modification in Bone Cancer Metastases

Chuan Yang[1],*
Zihan Deng[2],*
and Yueqi Chen[2],†

[1] Department of Biomedical Materials Science,
Third Military Medical University (Army Medical University),
Chongqing, People's Republic of China
[2] Department of Orthopedics, Southwest Hospital,
Third Military Medical University (Army Medical University),
Chongqing, People's Republic of China

Abstract

Bone is the most common site for metastasis in solid tumors, especially breast and prostate cancer. Bone metastasis, which causes a range of complications including bone pain, hypercalcemia, and fragility fracture, is a formidable challenge in cancer treatment and a leading cause of cancer mortality. N(6)-methyladenosine (m⁶A) is the most widespread and conserved posttranscriptional modification in cellular RNAs that regulates nearly all metabolism processes of RNAs, including RNA splicing, stability, nuclear export, and translation. Emerging evidence suggests that m⁶A is widely involved in cancer progression, such as tumorigenesis, proliferation, and metastasis. Although the specific mechanisms underlying bone metastasis remain unclear, increasing studies prove that m⁶A performs dual roles in bone metastasis *in situ* of

---

* Equal contributors.
† Corresponding Author's Email: chenyueqi1012@sina.com.

In: New Research on Bone Metastasis
Editor: Joseph Gerfried
ISBN: 979-8-88697-799-8
© 2023 Nova Science Publishers, Inc.

osteosarcoma (OS) and distant bone metastasis of prostate cancer (PCa) and breast cancer (BCa).

In the present chapter, we summarized recent research on m^{6}A modification and aimed to establish a theoretical basis for the application of m^{6}A in the early diagnosis and therapeutic implications of bone metastasis.

Keywords: N(6)-methyladenosine (m^{6}A) modification, bone metastasis, osteosarcoma (OS), prostate cancer (PCa), breast cancer (BCa)

Introduction

Bone metastasis is a prevalent complication of many cancers such as osteosarcoma (OS), prostate cancer (PCa), and breast cancer (BCa) that occurs in more than 1.5 million patients with cancer worldwide [1]. Bone metastasis is a gradual process in which tumor cells from the primary tumor undergo epithelial-to-mesenchymal transition (EMT) to invade the microvasculature and colonize in the bone marrow, and subsequently construct a cancer niche, ultimately disrupting normal bone homeostasis and gradually forming secondary cancer via the release of signals from the resorbed bone matrix [2]. Bone metastasis contributes to many bone-related events including bone pain, pathologic fracture, spinal compression, and hypercalcemia, resulting in elevated mortality in patients with advanced cancer. Treatment for bone metastasis includes chemoradiotherapy, endocrine therapy, and targeted therapy. Though these therapy options, especially bone-targeted agents (BTA) such as bisphosphonates and denosumab could effectively palliate morbidity associated with skeletal lesions, the median survival of patients with bone metastasis is still low [3]. It is therefore necessary to further probe the mechanisms of bone metastasis to prevent the progression of bone metastasis.

In recent years, epigenetic modification has become a major research hotspot, which can occur in different levels, including DNA, RNA, and histone modification, exerting a crucial role in regulating gene expression to affect cell development and differentiation [4-7]. Of note, the research of RNA modification is becoming the focused topic of epigenetics after DNA and histone modifications. Existing research has identified over 150 RNA modifications, of which m^{6}A is the most common modification that is widely distributed in messenger RNAs (mRNAs), transfer RNAs (tRNAs), ribosomal RNAs (rRNAs), non-coding RNAs (ncRNAs), as well as other types of RNAs

[8]. m⁶A modulates the alteration of RNA structure for initiating relevant functions such as nuclear translocation and RNA degradation. m⁶A modification is widespread in yeast, viruses, plants, drosophila, humans, and other mammals, and occurs in the adenosine base at the nitrogen-6 site of mRNAs [9]. The core sequence of m⁶A is RRm⁶ACH consensus sequence ([G/A/U] [G > A]m⁶AC [U > A > C]), located in the 3'untranslated regions (3'UTRs) adjacent to the stop codon of mRNAs
[10, 11]. Unlike other gene modifications, the discovery of demethylase FTO has determined that m⁶A RNA methylation is dynamically reversible, which is not only capable of serving as an epigenetic marker as DNA methylation and histone modification but also involved in modulating nearly all aspects of RNA metabolic processes, such as RNA splicing, nuclear export, localization, translation, and degradation [12-15].

m⁶A participates in multiple physiological processes such as neurophysiology, cellular differentiation, bone homeostasis, and so on. In contrast, disruption of m⁶A induces impaired gene expression and cellular function, which further leads to various diseases such as cancer, pathological bone diseases, and psychiatric disorders. While the specific mechanisms of bone metastasis remain to be completely elucidated, there is a growing body of evidence that m⁶A is widely involved in the progression of tumor-associated bone metastasis. In this chapter, we will focus on the recent progress of m⁶A during bone metastasis *in situ* such as OS and distant bone metastasis including PCa and BCa, and attempt to discuss the promising value of m⁶A in the clinical treatment of bone metastasis.

m⁶A RNA Methylation-Related Enzymes

m⁶A is one of the most ubiquitous intrinsic modifications of eukaryotic mRNAs, with abundance and function affected by interactions with methyltransferases, RNA-binding proteins, and demethylases [16, 17]. m⁶A is installed co-transcriptionally via a methyltransferase complex (MTC) which consists of three major components methyltransferase-like 3 (METTL3), methyltransferase-like 14 (METTL14), and Wilms tumor 1-associated protein (WTAP) [18]. As a stable heterodimer complex, METTL3-METTL14 is the essential component of MTC, playing a dramatic role in m⁶A deposition on nuclear RNAs [19]. METTL3 acts as a catalytic subunit, which is responsible for regulating alternative splicing of RNAs and transferring methyl groups to RNAs, while METTL14 assists in substrate binding and maintenance of the complex integrity [20, 21]. WTAP is responsible for the localization of METTL3-METTL14 complex to nuclear speckles and exerts a catalytic role in the activation of m^{6}A methyltransferase [18]. Besides, numerous accessory subunits of MTC have been identified, including RNA binding motif protein 15/15B (RBM15/15B), zinc finger CCCH-type containing 13 (ZC3H13), vir-like m^{6}A methyltransferase associated (VIRMA, also called KIAA1429), HAKAI, and methyltransferase-like protein 16 (METTL16).

Many studies have extensively documented that RBM15/15B is capable of mediating the transcriptional silencing of specific genes on the X chromosome via binding and recruiting m^{6}A MTC to specific sites in target mRNAs as well as long non-coding RNAs (lncRNAs) XIST [22]. As for ZC3H13/Flacc, it facilitates nuclear translocalization of the writer complex as well as primarily plays a crucial role in maintaining the stability of WTAP/Fl(2)d-RBM15/Nito interaction, which has been indicated to be involved in sex determination of drosophila [23]. Moreover, VIRMA is responsible for preferentially methylating mRNAs in 3`UTR and near-stop codon via interaction with MTC [22].

HAKAI is one of the core components of conserved m^{6}A MTC and has dramatic effects on interaction with other members and participation in sex-specific ways of m^{6}A modification [24]. Notably, METTL16, as a homologous protein of METTL3, installs m^{6}A in a different sequence and structure context to catalyze m^{6}A modifications in a variety of RNAs containing U6 small nuclear RNAs (snRNAs), lncRNAs, and pre-mRNAs through UAC(m^{6}A)GAGAA sequence in the bulge of a stem-loop [25, 26]. Meanwhile, METTL16 has been identified to exert a significant effect in the development of mouse embryos via modulating mRNAs level of S-adenosylmethionine (SAM) synthetase methionine adeno-syltransferase 2Z (MAT2Z) [27]. In addition, a heterodimeric complex formed by METTL5 and TRMT112 can transfer m^{6}A residues to 18S rRNAs, while ZCCHC4 is responsible for the diversion to 28S rRNAs and also interacts with a subset of mRNAs [28].

Demethylase can remove the methyl group of m^{6}A off RNAs and there are two common demethylases: fat mass and obesity-associated protein (FTO) and alkB homolog 5 (ALKBH5), which serve as members of the nonheme Fe (II)/α-ketoglutarate (α-KG)-dependent dioxygenases family exhibiting efficient oxidative demethylation activity of m^{6}A residues in RNAs [29, 30]. It is believed that m^{6}A in nuclear RNAs is the predominant physiological substrate of FTO, based on evidence that FTO is partially located on nuclear speckles. Besides, FTO makes effects on tremendous physiological activities including glycolysis and adipogenesis by removing m⁶A methylation in RNAs [31, 32]. Intriguingly, demethylation of FTO occurs preferentially at m⁶Am rather than m⁶A, which negatively modulates the stability of m⁶Am-containing mRNAs [33]. As another mammalian demethylase, ALKBH5 is also localized in the nucleus and significantly affects mRNAs nuclear export and mRNAs processing factor assembly in nuclear speckles, and is involved in the fertility impairment via aberrant spermatogenesis and apoptosis in mice [30]. Furthermore, ALKBH5-mediated erasure is associated with correct splicing and the ability to generate longer 3' -UTR mRNAs [34]. At present, few proteins exhibit demethylation activity and the mechanisms of selective identification of target transcripts with respect to FTO and ALKBH5 are still unclear. Indeed, acting as a conformational marker, m⁶A is capable of inducing diverse conformational outcomes in RNAs, thereby enabling demethylases to discriminate specific nucleotide sequences [35].

m⁶A "readers", as specific RNAs binding proteins, modulate the stability and translation of m⁶A-modified RNAs [36, 37]. The most common type of m⁶A "reader" proteins is the YT521-B homology (YTH) family, including YTHDC1, YTHDC2, YTHDF1, YTHDF2 and YTHDF3, which consists of the distinctive YTH domain as well as directly combine with m⁶A to modulate downstream targets [38-40]. Of these, YTHDC1 principally exists in the nucleus while the other "readers" are located in the cytoplasm. YTHDC1 is involved in mRNAs splicing through the recruitment of pre-mRNAs splicing factor SRSF3 and the blockade of SRSF10 mRNAs binding, eventually contributing to exon inclusion [41].

In addition, YTHDC1 facilitates RNAs binding to SRSF3 and NXF1 to mediate the nuclear export of m⁶A-containing mRNAs, thereby extending the potential utility of m⁶A modification [42]. It has been documented that YTHDC2 can selectively combine m⁶A to consensus motif, increasing the translation efficiency of target RNAs but decreasing their abundance [43]. YTHDF1 actively facilitates protein synthesis via interaction with the translation initiation complex, which ensures efficient protein production in a unified regulatory mechanism based on m⁶A [37]. As for YTHDF2, it is responsible for the selective recognition of m⁶A-modified mRNAs and ncRNAs via a conserved core motif G (m⁶A) C. And its carboxy-terminal domain combines with mRNAs, whereas the amino-terminal domain mediates the localization of YTHDF2-mRNA complex to cellular RNAs attenuation sites, inducing degradation of the transcripts [36].

Moreover, cooperating with YTHDF1, YTHDF3 plays an essential role in enhancing the translation efficiency of transcripts [44]. On the other hand,

YTHDF3 can directly interact with YTHDF2 to attenuate methylated mRNAs and facilitate transcript decay [45]. The second type of m^{6}A "reader" proteins is heterogeneous nuclear ribonucleoprotein (HNRNP) family, containing HNRNPA2B1, HNRNPC, and HNRNPG, which is in charge of modulating the maturation of RNAs substrates in the nucleus [46, 47]. Recent studies have shown that interacting with microRNAs (miRNAs) microprocessor complex protein DGCR8, HNRNPA2B1 makes a direct combination to m^{6}A sites, regulating primary miRNAs processing [46]. Meanwhile, an "m^{6}A-switch" mechanism has been proposed that m^{6}A may not directly combine with "readers" but change the structure of RNAs to promote RNAs binding to "readers", just as m^{6}A-modified RNAs bind to HNRNPA2B1, HNRNPC, and HNRNPG.

With accumulating researches focusing on m^{6}A methylation, other RNA-binding proteins have been found, including insulin-like growth factor 2 mRNA-binding proteins (IGF2BP), eukaryotic initiation factor 3 (EIF3), fragile X mental retardation 1 (FMR1), and leucine-rich pentatricopeptide repeat-containing (LRPPRC) [48, 49]. As a family of m^{6}A "readers" containing IGF2BP1-3, IGF2BPs are responsible for improving the stability of target transcripts as well as increasing their storage. The contrary function of IGF2BPs to YTHDF2 further indicates the core function of "reader" proteins in the regulation of transcript status and longevity. Additionally, directly bounding to a single 5'UTR m^{6}A modification, EIF3 recruits the 43S complex to initiate translation without the cap-binding factor EIF4E [50]. EIF3 also acts synergistically with METTL3 to improve the translation of certain mRNAs independently of the activity of m^{6}A "reader" proteins [51]. Notably, based on recent studies, FMR1 preferentially facilitates the nuclear export of m^{6}A-modified RNAs by CRM1, while the detailed bioactions of LRPPRC remain unclear [15, 52]. In fact, the potential number of m^{6}A "readers" is still large, and the modifications of m^{6}A rely on the "reader" proteins to fulfill biological functions, which are provided with an extensive research space.

In addition, accumulating evidence has suggested that m^{6}A participates in the regulation of dynamic balance of bone matrix as well as the formation of a complicated network in bone matrix metabolism. Therefore, the dysregulation of m^{6}A contributes to a variety of pathological bone diseases such as bone metastasis *in situ* of OS, and tumor-associated distant bone metastasis (Figure 1).

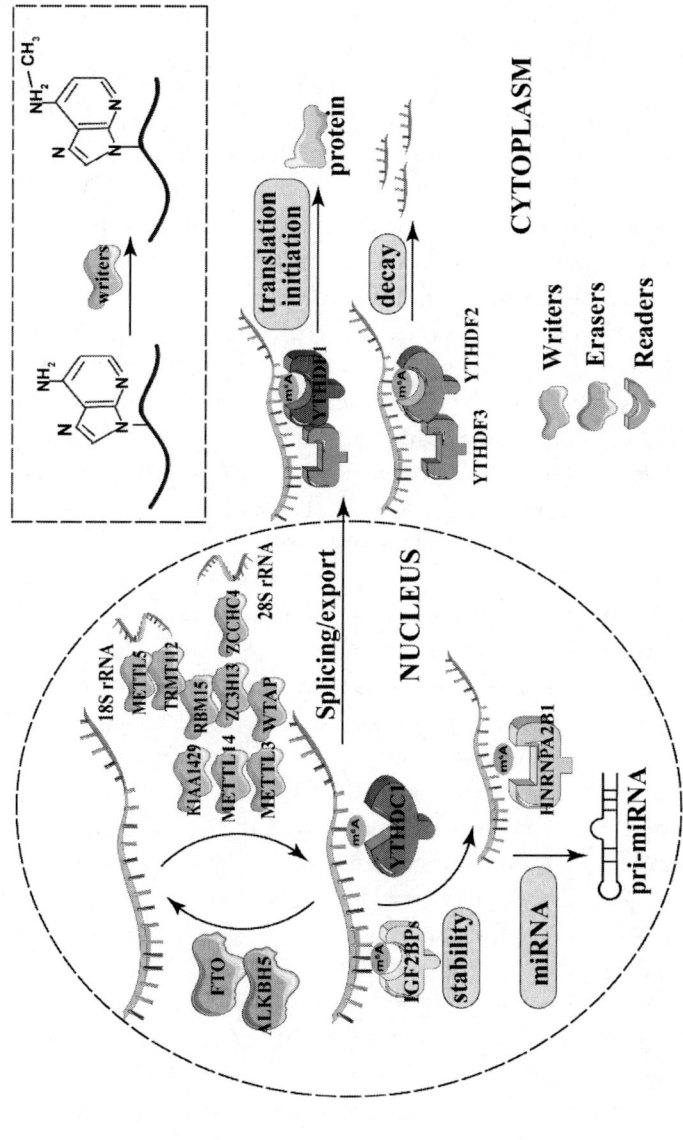

Figure 1. The biological functions of m⁶A regulators on RNAs. m⁶A modification is installed at specific sites in RNAs by methyltransferase complex or other independent methylases, and removed by specific demethylases, which maintains the reversible and dynamic equilibrium. RNA-binding proteins are the main implementers that regulate the metabolism processes of RNA including RNA splicing, nuclear export, translation, and degradation.

The Dual Role of m⁶A during Bone Metastasis *In Situ* of OS

OS is the most common primary malignant bone tumor in children, accounting for about 5% of pediatric tumors and 2.5% of pediatric malignancies, with a high fatality rate and invasiveness [53, 54]. Originating from osteoid and immature bone formed by malignant mesenchymal primitive transformed cells, OS is characterized by the production of bone-like tissue from spindle-shaped stromal cells [55, 56]. OS presents as a localized disease in more than 85% of patients, and its major growth site is the most active part of the bone, namely the metaphysis regions of long bones [57]. About 9% of patients with metastatic osteosarcoma have bone metastasis and 8% have bone and lung metastasis [58]. OS-induced bone lesions are characterized by osteolytic lesions, mainly mediated by osteoclasts and their bone-resorbing activity [59]. Bone-derived cytokines may promote OS growth, and OS cells are in turn able to release factors that stimulate osteoclast differentiation and activity, forming a vicious cycle that contributes to in-situ bone metastasis of OS to some extent [60]. The common therapeutic options for OS, consisting of surgery and chemotherapy, significantly improve the long-term survival (>70%) of patients with localized disease. However, the overall five-year survival rate of patients with metastatic tumors (<40%) remains unchanged over the past 30 years with the improvement of treatment regimens [53, 61]. The lack of effective treatment options for OS is partly due to the fact that the OS genome is highly disorganized and has a large tumor heterogeneity, which creates some difficult problems for OS therapy such as the identification of recurrent mutations and the mechanisms of recurrence [62, 63].

A growing number of research has demonstrated that m⁶A methylation and related regulators are involved in the occurrence, development, metastasis, and prognosis of OS. Transcriptome-wide m⁶A methylome data of osteosarcoma stem cells (OSCs) reported that METTL3, METTL14, and ALKBH5 are altered in OSCs, leading to different methylation levels in transcripts related to pluripotency of stem cells [64]. Furthermore, a comprehensive bioinformatic analysis demonstrated that high expression of HNRNPA2B1, KIAA1429, and YTHDF3 and low expression of METTL3, METTL14, FTO, and YTHDF2 were linked to poor prognosis in OS. m⁶A regulators may participate in OS progression via the humoral immune response and cell cycle pathways [65]. For instance, m⁶A plays a vital role in the advent and maintenance of OSCs by promoting the inactivation of BMP signaling and activation of canonical Wnt signaling [64].

Wujun Miao et al. found that total m⁶A level and relevant METTL3 expression are upregulated in human OS cell lines and facilitate cancer progression. Mechanically, METTL3 enhances the expression of lymphoid enhancer-binding factor 1 (LEF1), which activates the Wnt/β-catenin signaling pathway, ultimately promoting the carcinogenesis of OS [66]. GTP-binding protein (DRG) 1 is associated with the viability, migration, and colony formation abilities of OS cells. METTL3 also exerts a cancer-promoting effect by cooperating with ELAVL1 to increase DRG1 expression in an m⁶A-dependent manner [67]. In addition, METTL3 promotes proliferation and invasion of OS by increasing expression of ATPase family AAA domain containing 2 (ATAD2) and maintaining the stability of lncRNA DANCR and COPS5 transcript [68-70].

Furthermore, METTL3-mediated m⁶A modifications elevate the expression of circNRIP1, which upregulates FOXC2 by sponging miR-199a, exhibiting oncogenic roles in OS [71]. Qu's team found that METTL3 increases the m⁶A level of CCR4-NOT transcription complex subunit 7 (CNOT7) recognized by YTHDF1. YTHDF1 enhances the expression of CONT7 in an m⁶A-dependent manner, thereby promoting cell proliferation, migration and invasion of OS [72]. METTL3 also promotes the metastasis of OS cells by enhancing the expression of tumor necrosis factor receptor-associated factor 6 (TRAF6) and the specific mechanism still needs investigation [73]. Interestingly, METTL3 increases the m⁶A level of histone deacetylase 5 (HDAC5) to promote its expression, which reduces H3K9/K14ac on miR-142 promoter to suppress miR-142-5p expression, ultimately upregulating armadillo-repeat-containing 8 (ARMC8) level that facilitates OS cell proliferation. This study revealed the interplay between m⁶A and other epigenetic modifications, which helps investigate the important role of epigenetic reprogramming in OS progression [74].

Consistent with METTL3, METTL14 contributes to tumorigenesis and all-trans-retinoic acid resistance in OS. Mechanically, meningioma 1 (MN1) is methylated by METTL14 and subsequently recognized by IGF2BP2, which prevents MN1 mRNA degradation and enhances MN1 translation efficiency, leading to OS proliferation and metastasis [75]. WTAP expression is also upregulated in OS tissue and associated with poor prognosis in OS patients. WTAP reduces the stability of HMBOX1 mRNA depending in a YTHDF2-dependent manner, which alleviates the inhibitory effect of HMBOX1 on PI3K/AKT pathway and ultimately promotes OS growth and metastasis [76]. Furthermore, WTAP promotes methylation modifications and thereby enhances the stability of lncRNA FOXD2-AS1, which accelerates the migration, proliferation, and tumor growth of OS [77]. In addition to the above common m⁶A methyltransferase METTL3, METTL14, and WTAP, RBM15 is also closely correlated with OS metastasis formation and low survival rate of OS patients, serving as a useful and necessary biomarker for OS [78]. Mechanistically, RBM15 drives OS progression by facilitating m⁶A modification of aerobic glycolysis genes including hexokinase 2 (HK2), glucose-6-phosphate isomerase (GPI) and phosphoglycerate kinase 1 (PGK1). m⁶A methylation results in more stable mRNA and high expression of target genes, ultimately enhancing the glycolysis processes and activating OS progression [79].

Ye Yuan et al. found that ALKBH5 is downregulated in human OS and significantly inhibits the growth and motility of OS cells. Mechanistically, Yes-associated protein 1 (YAP) is an oncogene that plays an important role in multiple tumor development including OS. On the one hand, ALKBH5 maintains the stability of pre-miR-181b-1 by inhibiting YTHDF2-mediated RNA degradation, which targets and downregulates YAP expression. On the other hand, ALKBH5 suppresses the YTHDF1-mediated translation of YAP mRNA, thereby suppressing OS progression [80]. Zechuan Yang et al. also proved that ALKBH5 upregulation could reduce m⁶A mRNA levels in human OS cells, thereby inhibiting cell proliferation and leading to cell apoptosis and cycle arrest. ALKBH5-mediated demethylation blocks YTHDF2 from recognizing m⁶A-modified suppressors of cytokine signaling 3 (SOCS3) mRNA and subsequent decay. As the negative regulator of STAT3, SOCS3 inactivates STAT3 pathway and therefore inhibits cell proliferation and survival of OS [81]. Three-phosphoinositide-dependent protein kinase 1(PDPK1) was reported to activate AKT/mTOR pathway and thereby promoted the malignant progression of OS. Dong Cao et al. found that YTHDC1 promotes cell growth, migration and EMT in OS by stabilizing PDPK1 mRNA via m⁶A-dependent regulation [82]. YTHDF3 expression is also upregulated in OS samples and accelerates tumor growth by enhancing PGK1 mRNA stability in an m⁶A-dependent manner [83].

However, much research has shown almost opposite results regarding the role of m⁶A in OS. Tripartite motif-containing protein 7 (TRIM7), an E3 ubiquitin ligase that modulates OS cell invasion, migration, and chemoresistance through ubiquitination of BRMS1, is downregulated via a METTL3-YTHDF2-dependent manner [84]. In addition, METTL14 also inhibits OS cell viability and proliferation and promotes OS cell apoptosis. The anti-tumor properties of METTL14 are achieved by the activation of caspase-3, the most important terminal shear enzyme in cell apoptosis [85].

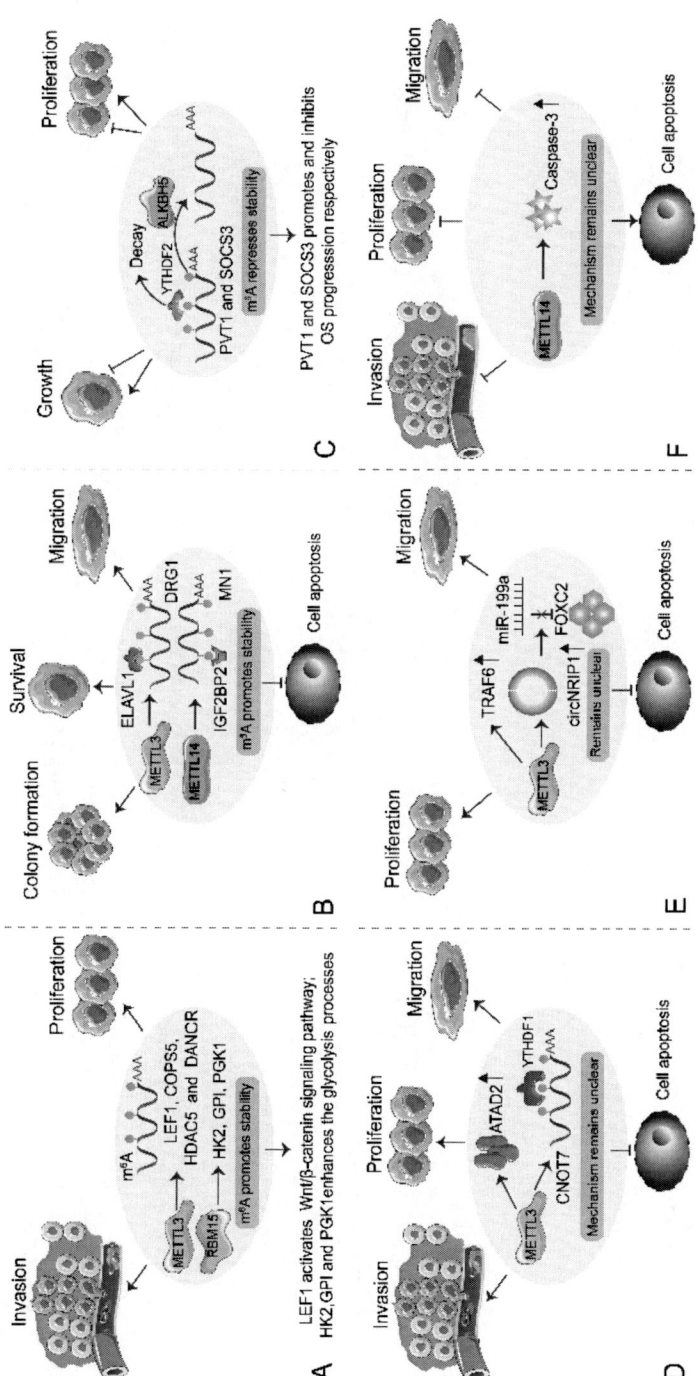

Figure 2. (Continued).

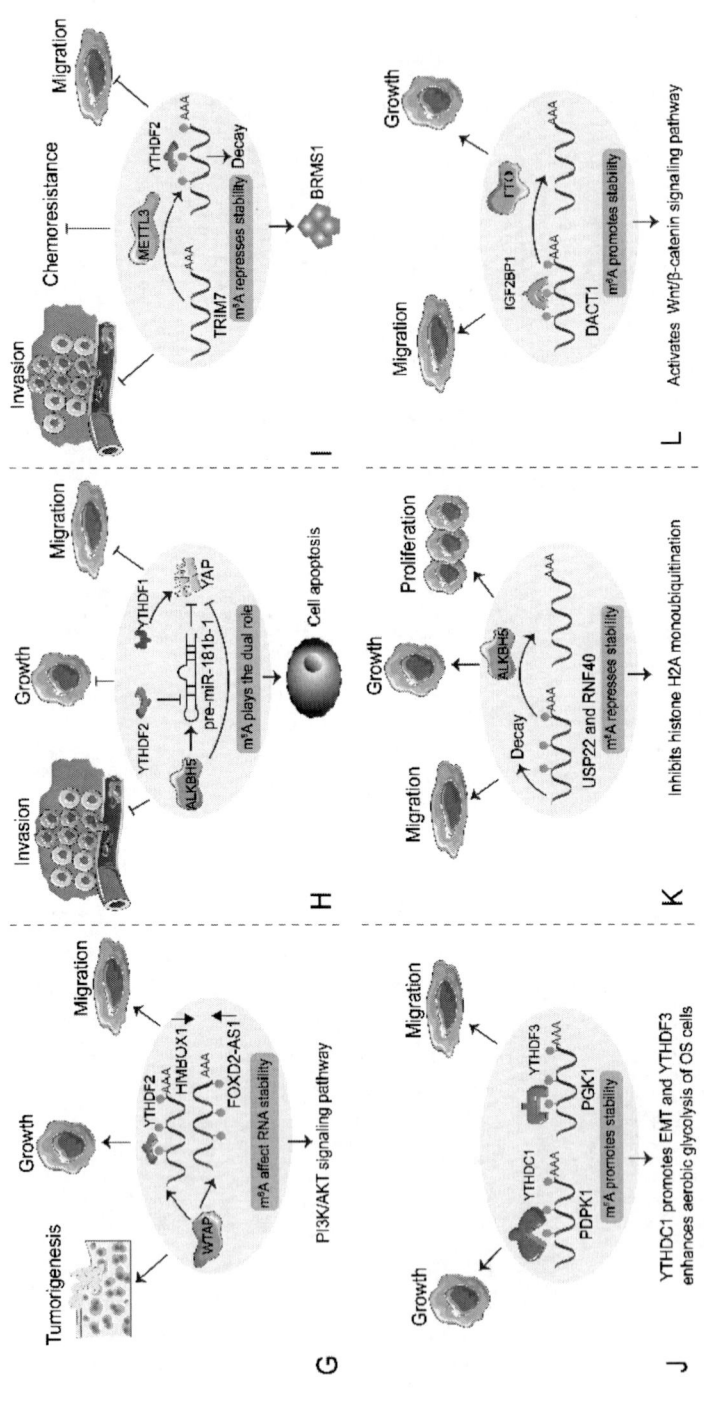

Figure 2. The role of m⁶A in osteosarcoma (OS). m⁶A modification plays a dual role in the progression of OS. On the one hand, m⁶A promotes OS progression by upregulating oncogene expression and downregulating tumor suppressor gene expression. On the other hand, m⁶A modification hampers OS pathogenesis by inhibiting oncogene expression and enhancing tumor suppressor gene expression. This is an m⁶A-based regulatory network that consists of methyltransferase, demethylases, RNA-binding proteins, downstream genes, and signaling pathways.

Manjeet K Rao et al. proved that ALKBH5-mediated demethylation upregulates expression of the histone deubiquitinase USP22 and the ubiquitin ligase RNF40, which block histone H2A monoubiquitination and induction of key protumorigenic genes, leading to unchecked cell-cycle progression, incessant replication, and DNA repair [62]. ALKBH5 also promotes OS cell proliferation *in vitro* and tumor growth *in vivo* by increasing the expression of PVT1 via a YTHDF2-dependent manner [86]. Dapper1/Frodo1 (DACT1), a homologue of Dapper, is a novel inhibitor of the WNT/β-catenin signaling that plays an anticarcinogenic role in many different forms of cancer [87, 88]. Dongming Lv et al. found that FTO reduces the m^{6}A level of DACT1 transcript, which blocks the recognition of IGF2BP1 to DACT1 and reduces DACT1 stability, further activating the Wnt signaling pathway and promoting OS growth and metastasis [89].

Based on the above experimental results, m^{6}A plays a dual role in OS progression, presumably due to its wide distribution in many key pluripotency and developmental regulators. It is a complex regulatory network consisting of m^{6}A, m^{6}A regulators, and various target genes that connects multiple mRNAs, lncRNAs, miRNAs, histone modifications, and signaling pathways, ultimately driving the cell in a particular direction. Within this complex m^{6}A regulatory network, m^{6}A-related lncRNA expression has been widely used as a prognostic biomarker of OS, independent of other clinical characteristics. As a functional molecule distinct from mRNA, lncRNA is a better proxy for disease status than a template for protein synthesis. Highly specific expression patterns are strongly associated with immune infiltration, cancer microenvironment, and immune-associated genes, which can help predict patient outcomes and guide the application of immunotherapeutic drugs to OS patients (Figure 2) [90, 91].

The Biregulatory Role of m^{6}A in Tumor-Associated Distant Bone Metastasis

PCa is one of the most common malignancies of the male genitourinary system that serves as the secondary fatal cause in male patients with cancer worldwide. PCa tends to metastasize to bone, with approximately 80% of metastatic PCa cells spreading to the bones, particularly the vertebrae [92]. Indeed, appropriately 90% of PCa patients develop bone metastasis and 3% of patients are still alive at five years [93]. However, existing treatments for PCa-associated bone metastasis are still inadequate. It is useful for disease control to elucidate the specific molecular mechanisms underlying PCa-associated bone metastasis. METTL3 expression is upregulated in PCa tissue, especially in PCa tissue with bone metastasis compared to normal prostate tissues. High expression of METTL3 is positively associated with the prognosis of PCa with advanced bone metastases, which reveals the significant role of m^{6}A in bone metastasis of PCa [94].

Type I collagen, the most common bone protein, binds to cancer cells and promotes their targeted migration to the bone. Functional assays demonstrated that METTL3 upregulates the expression of Integrin β1 (ITGB1) in an m^{6}A-HuR-dependent manner, which enhances the ability of PCa cells adhesion to Collagen I and tumor cell motility, eventually promoting bone metastasis of PCa [94]. Yu Zhao's group identified four credible m^{6}A sites on lncRNA NEAT1-1 that are related to PCa-associated bone metastasis and could be a powerful predictor of the patient outcome. Mechanistically, the m^{6}A methylation modifications on lncRNA NEAT1-1 contribute to the phosphorylation of Pol II ser2 in the promoter of RUNX2 by facilitating binding between CYCLINL1 and CDK19, which ultimately induces metastasis of cancer cells to the bone [95]. Prostate cancer-associated transcript 6 (PCAT6), as a common oncogene in non-small-cell lung cancer, is also upregulated in PCa tissues with bone metastasis and promotes PCa cell invasion, migration, and proliferation. METTL3-mediated m^{6}A modification promotes the recognition and binding of methylated PCAT6 by IGF2BP2, which maintains the stability of PCAT6 and enhances its expression. Subsequently, PCAT6 participates in the formation of the PCAT6/IGF2BP2/IGF1R complex to enhance IGF1R mRNA stability, which contributes to IGF1R upregulation and promotes bone metastasis in PCa [96]. Lnc-NAP1L6 has been proven to act as an oncogene in PCa that could promote cell migration and β-catenin expression [97].

Recent studies have found that lnc-NAP1L6 is overexpressed in PCa-associated bone metastasis cell lines compared with normal cell lines and may function in PCa-associated bone metastasis. The mechanism assays demonstrated that the METTL14/METTL3 complex increases the m^{6}A methylation levels of NAP1L2 transcript, after which the RNA-binding protein HNRNPC is recruited to m^{6}A-modified NAP1L2 by lncNAP1L6 to maintain its stability. NAP1L2 enhances the transcription of MMP2 and MMP9 by interacting with YY1, leading to the activation of the MMP signaling pathway and promoting bone metastasis of PCa [98].

Table 1. The role of m⁶A methylation in bone metastasis

m⁶A regulators	Target RNA	Biological functions on target RNA	Role of m⁶A in cancer	References
METTL3	LEF1	stability	promotes the cell proliferation, migration, and invasion ability of OS cells	[66]
METTL3	DRG1	stability	promotes growth, migration, and colony formation in OS	[67]
METTL3	ATAD2	unclear	promotes proliferation and invasion of OS	[68]
METTL3	DANCR	stability	promotes OS cell proliferation, migration, and invasion	[69]
METTL3	COPS5	stability	promotes proliferation and migration of OS	[70]
METTL3	circNRIP1	unclear	promotes proliferation and migration of OS	[71]
METTL3	CNOT7	unclear	promotes proliferation, migration, and invasion of OS cells	[72]
METTL3	TRAF6	unclear	promotes OS cell migration, invasion, epithelial-mesenchymal transition (EMT), and tumorigenic and metastatic activities	[73]
METTL3	HDAC5	stability	facilitates the malignant proliferation of OS cells	[74]
METTL14	MN1	stability and translation	promotes tumorigenicity and all-trans-retinoic acid resistance in OS	[75]
WTAP	HMBOX1	stability	promotes OS growth and metastasis	[76]
WTAP	FOXD2-AS1	stability	accelerates the migration, proliferation, and tumor growth of OS	[77]
RBM15	HK2, GPI, PGK1	stability	enhances the glycolysis processes and activates OS progression	[79]
ALKBH5	pre-miR-181b-1 and YAP	stability and translation	promotes OS cell growth, migration, and invasion, and inhibits cell apoptosis	[80]
ALKBH5	SOCS3	stability	maintains cell proliferation and survival of OS	[81]
YTHDC1	PDPK1	stability	promotes cell growth, migration, and EMT in OS	[82]
YTHDF3	PGK1	stability	promotes the proliferation and aerobic glycolysis of OS cells *in vitro*, and accelerates the tumor growth *in vivo*	[83]
METTL3	TRIM7	stability	inhibits OS cell invasion, migration, and chemoresistance	[84]
METTL14	caspase-3	unclear	reduces the proliferation, migration, and invasion and promotes apoptosis of OS cells	[85]
ALKBH5	USP22 and RNF40	stability	inhibits OS growth and progression	[62]
ALKBH5	PVT1	stability	inhibits OS cell proliferation *in vitro* and tumor growth *in vivo*	[86]
FTO	DACT1	stability	inhibits OS growth and metastasis	[89]

Table 1. (Continued)

m⁶A regulators	Target RNA	Biological functions on target RNA	Role of m⁶A in cancer	References
METTL3	ITGB1	stability	enhances the ability of PCa cell adhesion to Collagen I and tumor cell motility, and promotes bone metastasis of PCa	[94]
METTL3	NEAT1-1	unclear	induces PCa cell metastasis to lung and bone	[95]
METTL3	PCAT6	stability	promotes PCa-associated bone metastasis	[96]
METTL14/ METTL3	NAP1L2	stability	activates MMP signaling pathway and promotes bone metastasis of PCa	[98]
YTHDF2	FGF14-AS2	stability	promotes osteoclast differentiation and osteolytic metastasis of BCa	[101]

Bone is also the most common organ of breast cancer (BCa) metastasis that is affected in more than 70% of patients with metastatic breast cancer (MBC) [99]. The lncRNA FGF14-AS2 has been proven to be an important suppressor that inhibits BCa metastasis by serving as a competing endogenous RNA (ceRNA) for miR-370-3p [100]. Recent studies found that YTHDF2 expression is increased in BCa and promotes osteoclast differentiation and osteolytic metastasis of BCa by mediating RNA degradation of FGF14-AS2. FGF14-AS2 inhibits the assembly of the eIF4E/eIF4G complex and the phosphorylation of eIF4E, which suppresses the translation of RUNX2 and ultimately reduces the transcription of RANKL, a critical regulator of osteoclast differentiation (Table 1) [101].

Conclusion and Future Perspectives

Although the therapy options for bone metastases have changed significantly over the past decade with the adoption of new therapeutic strategies, the prognosis remains poor, mainly due to the heterogeneity of bone metastasis and drug resistance. m⁶A, as a novel posttranscriptional modification, plays an important role in the process of bone metastasis by widely affecting RNA metabolism and translation. As mentioned above, m⁶A performs completely different functions in different cancers, including tumor inhibition or promotion. On the one hand, abnormal m⁶A modification promotes the progression of bone metastasis via the upregulation of oncogenes or the silencing of anti-oncogene. On the other hand, m⁶A can inhibit bone metastasis via the opposite regulation. The dual role is due to the wide distribution of m⁶A in abundant transcripts and multiple RNA-binding proteins that mediate different effects in RNA metabolism and translation. There is a different expressed pattern of m⁶A modification in the process of bone metastasis. Therefore, the construction of m⁶A-related regulators and transcripts (including mRNAs, lncRNAs, miRNAs, and so on) pair prognostic signature and prediction of the immune landscape may provide a rationale for research on bone metastasis and guide the chemotherapeutics strategies for patients.

Bone metastases are constantly classified into three types: osteolytic, osteoblastic, and mixed [102]. Osteolytic bone metastases usually occur in breast cancer, lung cancer, and renal cancer, while the osteoblastic disease is associated with prostate cancer [103]. The release of tumor-derived factors that stimulate osteoclast formation and osteoclast differentiation is the main cause of the formation of the aforementioned bone metastasis phenotypes. Therefore, elucidating the molecular mechanisms of osteogenic and osteoclast differentiation may be beneficial for the identification of effective potential targets and stratified management of patients with bone metastasis. m⁶A modification has been proved to be widely present in transcripts that regulate lineage, precisely determining the differentiation of osteoclasts and osteoblasts [8]. Combining studies of m⁶A in cell differentiation and bone metastasis is helpful for a more comprehensive understanding of the mechanisms of bone metastasis and improved BCa prognosis.

Epigenetic modification such as DNA methylation has been widely applied in cancer treatment. Azacytidine and decitabine, as the inhibitors of DNA methylation, hold up fairly well in anticancer treatment including pancreatic cancer, bladder cancer, breast cancer, and so on. As mentioned above, aberrant expression of m⁶A regulators is closely associated with the progression of tumor-related bone metastasis and the prognosis of cancer patients. Therefore, m⁶A regulators may be also potential and promising biological targets for the treatment of bone metastasis. Indeed, current studies have identified more than 20 m⁶A modification regulators, but only a few of them could serve as ideal targets for cancer molecular targeting therapy. Meanwhile, novel drug development related to m⁶A regulators is slow and costly. Although many m⁶A activators such as curcumin and saikosaponin as well as inhibitors including betaine and quercetin have been reported, none of them has been approved to treat bone metastasis due to the poor target specificity and safety. Thus, the development of novel m⁶A-related drugs targeting bone metastasis is an important and prospective research field.

m^{6}A is a significant epigenetic modification that regulates bone metastasis by triggering the key molecules and signaling pathways. However, there are many limitations in related studies:

- Virtually all of research has reported the association between m^{6}A regulators and bone metastasis, but the underlying mechanisms remain unclear, which restricts the construction of m^{6}A-regulatory network.
- The "reader" proteins are the main implementers in the m^{6}A-mediated biological function and their aberrant expression leads to severe metabolic disorders of RNA. However, existing studies focus on YTH family, while ignoring the less studied m^{6}A readers, such as EIF3, FMR1, and HNRNP family.
- Many bioinformatic analyses that focus on the association between m^{6}A regulators and the prognosis of patients have shown different and even opposite results, which may be limited due to the insufficient sample size and many interference factors, leading to rampant random associations.

Therefore, we need more investigation to explore the specific association between m^{6}A regulators and the progression of bone metastasis.

In conclusion, given the crucial effects of m^{6}A on bone metastasis, it is of great significance to search for more novel m^{6}A regulators that could be used as potential diagnostic and therapeutic targets. More studies are needed to develop effective activators or inhibitors of m^{6}A that block the progression of bone metastasis.

References

[1] Weilbaecher, K. N., Guise, T. A., McCauley, L. K. (2011) Cancer to bone: a fatal attraction. *Nature Reviews. Cancer* 11:411-425.

[2] Clézardin, P., Coleman, R., Puppo, M., Ottewell, P., Bonnelye, E., Paycha, F., Confavreux, C. B., Holen, I. (2021) Bone metastasis: mechanisms, therapies, and biomarkers. *Physiological Reviews* 101:797-855.

[3] Selvaggi, G., Scagliotti, G. V. (2005) Management of bone metastases in cancer: a review. *Critical Reviews in Oncology/Hematology* 56:365-378.

[4] Kohli, R. M., Zhang, Y. (2013) TET enzymes, TDG and the dynamics of DNA demethylation. *Nature* 502:472-479.

[5] Litt, M. D., Simpson, M., Gaszner, M., Allis, C. D., Felsenfeld, G. (2001) Correlation between histone lysine methylation and developmental changes at the chicken beta-globin locus. *Science (New York, N.Y.)* 293:2453-2455.

[6] Roignant, J. Y., Soller, M. (2017) m(6)A in mRNA: An Ancient Mechanism for Fine-Tuning Gene Expression. *Trends in Genetics : TIG* 33:380-390.

[7] Helm, M., Motorin, Y. (2017) Detecting RNA modifications in the epitranscriptome: predict and validate. *Nature Reviews. Genetics* 18:275-291.

[8] Yang, C., Dong, Z., Ling, Z., Chen, Y. (2022) The crucial mechanism and therapeutic implication of RNA methylation in bone pathophysiology. *Ageing Research Reviews* 79:101641.

[9] Wei, C. M., Gershowitz, A., Moss, B. (1975) Methylated nucleotides block 5' terminus of HeLa cell messenger RNA. *Cell* 4:379-386.

[10] Dominissini, D., Moshitch-Moshkovitz, S., Schwartz, S., Salmon-Divon, M., Ungar, L., Osenberg, S., Cesarkas, K., Jacob-Hirsch, J., Amariglio, N., Kupiec, M., Sorek, R., Rechavi, G. (2012) Topology of the human and mouse m6A RNA methylomes revealed by m6A-seq. *Nature* 485:201-206.

[11] Meyer, K. D., Saletore, Y., Zumbo, P., Elemento, O., Mason, C. E., Jaffrey, S. R. (2012) Comprehensive analysis of mRNA methylation reveals enrichment in 3' UTRs and near stop codons. *Cell* 149:1635-1646.

[12] Haussmann, I. U., Bodi, Z., Sanchez-Moran, E., Mongan, N. P., Archer, N., Fray, R. G., Soller, M. (2016) m(6)A potentiates Sxl alternative pre-mRNA splicing for robust Drosophila sex determination. *Nature* 540:301-304.

[13] Guo, M., Liu, X., Zheng, X., Huang, Y., Chen, X. (2017) m(6)A RNA Modification Determines Cell Fate by Regulating mRNA Degradation. *Cellular Reprogramming* 19:225-231.

[14] Yu, J., Chen, M., Huang, H., Zhu, J., Song, H., Zhu, J., Park, J., Ji, S. J. (2018) Dynamic m6A modification regulates local translation of mRNA in axons. *Nucleic Acids Research* 46:1412-1423.

[15] Edens, B. M., Vissers, C., Su, J., Arumugam, S., Xu, Z., Shi, H., Miller, N., Rojas Ringeling, F., Ming, G. L., He, C., Song, H., Ma, Y. C. (2019) FMRP Modulates Neural Differentiation through m(6)A-Dependent mRNA Nuclear Export. *Cell Reports* 28:845-854.e845.

[16] Panneerdoss, S., Eedunuri, V. K., Yadav, P., Timilsina, S., Rajamanickam, S., Viswanadhapalli, S., Abdelfattah, N., Onyeagucha, B. C., Cui, X., Lai, Z., Mohammad, T. A., Gupta, Y. K., Huang, T. H., Huang, Y., Chen, Y., Rao, M. K. (2018) Cross-talk among writers, readers, and erasers of m(6)A regulates cancer growth and progression. *Science Advances* 4:eaar8263.

[17] Shi, H., Wei, J., He, C. (2019) Where, When, and How: Context-Dependent Functions of RNA Methylation Writers, Readers, and Erasers. *Molecular cell* 74:640-650.

[18] Ping, X. L., Sun, B. F., Wang, L., Xiao, W., Yang, X., Wang, W. J., et al (2014) Mammalian WTAP is a regulatory subunit of the RNA N6-methyladenosine methyltransferase. *Cell Research* 24:177-189.

[19] Liu, J., Yue, Y., Han, D., Wang, X., Fu, Y., Zhang, L., et al. (2014) A METTL3-METTL14 complex mediates mammalian nuclear RNA N6-adenosine methylation. *Nature Chemical Biology* 10:93-95.

[20] Feng, Z., Li, Q., Meng, R., Yi, B., Xu, Q. (2018) METTL3 regulates alternative splicing of MyD88 upon the lipopolysaccharide-induced inflammatory response in human dental pulp cells. *Journal of Cellular and Molecular Medicine* 22:2558-2568.

[21] Wang, X., Feng, J., Xue, Y., Guan, Z., Zhang, D., Liu, Z., Gong, Z., Wang, Q., Huang, J., Tang, C., Zou, T., Yin, P. (2016) Structural basis of N(6)-adenosine methylation by the METTL3-METTL14 complex. *Nature* 534:575-578.

[22] Patil, D. P., Chen, C. K., Pickering, B. F., Chow, A., Jackson, C., Guttman, M., Jaffrey, S. R. (2016) m(6)A RNA methylation promotes XIST-mediated transcriptional repression. *Nature* 537:369-373.

[23] Knuckles, P., Lence, T., Haussmann, I. U., Jacob, D., Kreim, N., Carl, S. H., et al. (2018) Zc3h13/Flacc is required for adenosine methylation by bridging the mRNA-binding factor Rbm15/Spenito to the m(6)A machinery component Wtap/Fl(2)d. *Genes & Development* 32:415-429.

[24] Bawankar, P., Lence, T., Paolantoni, C., Haussmann, I. U., Kazlauskiene, M., Jacob, D., Heidelberger, J. B., Richter, F. M., Nallasivan, M. P., Morin, V., Kreim, N., Beli, P., Helm, M., Jinek, M., Soller, M., Roignant, J. Y. (2021) Hakai is required for stabilization of core components of the m(6)A mRNA methylation machinery. *Nature Communications* 12:3778.

[25] Doxtader, K. A., Wang, P., Scarborough, A. M., Seo, D., Conrad, N. K., Nam, Y. (2018) Structural Basis for Regulation of METTL16, an S-Adenosylmethionine Homeostasis Factor. *Molecular Cell* 71:1001-1011.e1004.

[26] Pendleton, K. E., Chen, B., Liu, K., Hunter, O. V., Xie, Y., Tu, B. P., Conrad, N. K. (2017) The U6 snRNA m(6)A Methyltransferase METTL16 Regulates SAM Synthetase Intron Retention. *Cell* 169:824-835.e814.

[27] Mendel, M., Chen, K. M., Homolka, D., Gos, P., Pandey, R. R., McCarthy, A. A., Pillai, R. S. (2018) Methylation of Structured RNA by the m(6)A Writer METTL16 Is Essential for Mouse Embryonic Development. *Molecular Cell* 71:986-1000.e1011.

[28] Ma, H., Wang, X., Cai, J., Dai, Q., Natchiar, S. K., Lv, R., Chen, K., Lu, Z., Chen, H., Shi, Y. G., Lan, F., Fan, J., Klaholz, B. P., Pan, T., Shi, Y., He, C. (2019) N(6-)Methyladenosine methyltransferase ZCCHC4 mediates ribosomal RNA methylation. *Nature Chemical Biology* 15:88-94.

[29] Jia, G., Fu, Y., Zhao, X., Dai, Q., Zheng, G., Yang, Y., Yi, C., Lindahl, T., Pan, T., Yang, Y. G., He, C. (2011) N6-methyladenosine in nuclear RNA is a major substrate of the obesity-associated FTO. *Nature Chemical Biology* 7:885-887.

[30] Zheng, G., Dahl, J. A., Niu, Y., Fedorcsak, P., Huang, C. M., Li, C. J., et al. (2013) ALKBH5 is a mammalian RNA demethylase that impacts RNA metabolism and mouse fertility. *Molecular Cell* 49:18-29.

[31] Qing, Y., Dong, L., Gao, L., Li, C., Li, Y., Han, L., et al. (2021) R-2-hydroxyglutarate attenuates aerobic glycolysis in leukemia by targeting the FTO/m(6)A/PFKP/LDHB axis. *Molecular Cell* 81:922-939.e929.

[32] Wang, L., Song, C., Wang, N., Li, S., Liu, Q., Sun, Z., Wang, K., Yu, S. C., Yang, Q. (2020) NADP modulates RNA m(6)A methylation and adipogenesis via enhancing FTO activity. *Nature Chemical Biology* 16:1394-1402.

[33] Mauer, J., Luo, X., Blanjoie, A., Jiao, X., Grozhik, A. V., Patil, D. P., Linder, B., Pickering, B. F., Vasseur, J. J., Chen, Q., Gross, S. S., Elemento, O., Debart, F., Kiledjian, M., Jaffrey, S. R. (2017) Reversible methylation of m(6)A(m) in the 5' cap controls mRNA stability. *Nature* 541:371-375.

[34] Tang, C., Klukovich, R., Peng, H., Wang, Z., Yu, T., Zhang, Y., Zheng, H., Klungland, A., Yan, W. (2018) ALKBH5-dependent m6A demethylation controls splicing and stability of long 3'-UTR mRNAs in male germ cells. *Proceedings of the National Academy of Sciences of the United States of America* 115:E325-e333.

[35] Zou, S., Toh, J. D., Wong, K. H., Gao, Y. G., Hong, W., Woon, E. C. (2016) N(6)-Methyladenosine: a conformational marker that regulates the substrate specificity of human demethylases FTO and ALKBH5. *Sci Rep* 6:25677.

[36] Wang, X., Lu, Z., Gomez, A., Hon, G. C., Yue, Y., Han, D., Fu, Y., Parisien, M., Dai, Q., Jia, G., Ren, B., Pan, T., He, C. (2014) N6-methyladenosine-dependent regulation of messenger RNA stability. *Nature* 505:117-120.

[37] Wang, X., Zhao, B. S., Roundtree, I. A., Lu, Z., Han, D., Ma, H., Weng, X., Chen, K., Shi, H., He, C. (2015) N(6)-methyladenosine Modulates Messenger RNA Translation Efficiency. *Cell* 161:1388-1399.

[38] Luo, S., Tong, L. (2014) Molecular basis for the recognition of methylated adenines in RNA by the eukaryotic YTH domain. *Proceedings of the National Academy of Sciences of the United States of America* 111:13834-13839.

[39] Xu, C., Wang, X., Liu, K., Roundtree, I. A., Tempel, W., Li, Y., Lu, Z., He, C., Min, J. (2014) Structural basis for selective binding of m6A RNA by the YTHDC1 YTH domain. *Nature Chemical Biology* 10:927-929.

[40] Kasowitz, S. D., Ma, J., Anderson, S. J., Leu, N. A., Xu, Y., Gregory, B. D., Schultz, R. M., Wang, P. J. (2018) Nuclear m6A reader YTHDC1 regulates alternative polyadenylation and splicing during mouse oocyte development. *PLoS Genetics* 14:e1007412.

[41] Xiao, W., Adhikari, S., Dahal, U., Chen, Y. S., Hao, Y. J., Sun, B. F., Sun, H. Y., Li, A., Ping, X. L., Lai, W. Y., Wang, X., Ma, H. L., Huang, C. M., Yang, Y., Huang, N., Jiang, G. B., Wang, H. L., Zhou, Q., Wang, X. J., Zhao, Y. L., Yang, Y. G. (2016) Nuclear m(6)A Reader YTHDC1 Regulates mRNA Splicing. *Molecular Cell* 61:507-519.

[42] Roundtree, I. A., Luo, G. Z., Zhang, Z., Wang, X., Zhou, T., Cui, Y., Sha, J., Huang, X., Guerrero, L., Xie, P., He, E., Shen, B., He, C. (2017) YTHDC1 mediates nuclear export of N(6)-methyladenosine methylated mRNAs. *eLife* 6.

[43] Hsu, P. J., Zhu, Y., Ma, H., Guo, Y., Shi, X., Liu, Y., Qi, M., Lu, Z., Shi, H., Wang, J., Cheng, Y., Luo, G., Dai, Q., Liu, M., Guo, X., Sha, J., Shen, B., He, C. (2017) Ythdc2 is an N(6)-methyladenosine binding protein that regulates mammalian spermatogenesis. *Cell Research* 27:1115-1127.

[44] Li, A., Chen, Y. S., Ping, X. L., Yang, X., Xiao, W., Yang, Y., Sun, H. Y., Zhu, Q., Baidya, P., Wang, X., Bhattarai, D. P., Zhao, Y. L., Sun, B. F., Yang, Y. G. (2017)

Cytoplasmic m(6)A reader YTHDF3 promotes mRNA translation. *Cell Research* 27:444-447.

[45] Shi, H., Wang, X., Lu, Z., Zhao, B. S., Ma, H., Hsu, P. J., Liu, C., He, C. (2017) YTHDF3 facilitates translation and decay of N(6)-methyladenosine-modified RNA. *Cell Research* 27:315-328.

[46] Alarcón, C. R., Goodarzi, H., Lee, H., Liu, X., Tavazoie, S., Tavazoie, S. F. (2015) HNRNPA2B1 Is a Mediator of m(6)A-Dependent Nuclear RNA Processing Events. *Cell* 162:1299-1308.

[47] Liu, N., Dai, Q., Zheng, G., He, C., Parisien, M., Pan, T. (2015) N(6)-methyladenosine-dependent RNA structural switches regulate RNA-protein interactions. *Nature* 518:560-564.

[48] Huang, H., Weng, H., Sun, W., Qin, X., Shi, H., Wu, H., et al. (2018) Recognition of RNA N(6)-methyladenosine by IGF2BP proteins enhances mRNA stability and translation. *Nature Cell Biology* 20:285-295.

[49] Zhang, F., Kang, Y., Wang, M., Li, Y., Xu, T., Yang, W., Song, H., Wu, H., Shu, Q., Jin, P. (2018) Fragile X mental retardation protein modulates the stability of its m6A-marked messenger RNA targets. *Human Molecular Genetics* 27:3936-3950.

[50] Meyer, K. D., Patil, D. P., Zhou, J., Zinoviev, A., Skabkin, M. A., Elemento, O., Pestova, T. V., Qian, S. B., Jaffrey, S. R. (2015) 5' UTR m(6)A Promotes Cap-Independent Translation. *Cell* 163:999-1010.

[51] Choe, J., Lin, S., Zhang, W., Liu, Q., Wang, L., Ramirez-Moya, J., Du, P., Kim, W., Tang, S., Sliz, P., Santisteban, P., George, R. E., Richards, W. G., Wong, K. K., Locker, N., Slack, F. J., Gregory, R. I. (2018) mRNA circularization by METTL3-eIF3h enhances translation and promotes oncogenesis. *Nature* 561:556-560.

[52] Arguello, A. E., DeLiberto, A. N., Kleiner, R. E. (2017) RNA Chemical Proteomics Reveals the N(6)-Methyladenosine (m(6)A)-Regulated Protein-RNA Interactome. *Journal of the American Chemical Society* 139:17249-17252.

[53] Kansara, M., Teng, M. W., Smyth, M. J., Thomas, D. M. (2014) Translational biology of osteosarcoma. *Nature Reviews. Cancer* 14:722-735.

[54] Duong, L. M., Richardson, L. C. (2013) Descriptive epidemiology of malignant primary osteosarcoma using population-based registries, United States, 1999-2008. *Journal of Registry Management* 40:59-64.

[55] Chen, C., Xie, L., Ren, T., Huang, Y., Xu, J., Guo, W. (2021) Immunotherapy for osteosarcoma: Fundamental mechanism, rationale, and recent breakthroughs. *Cancer Letters* 500:1-10.

[56] Chen, Y., Miao, L., Lin, H., Zhuo, Z., He, J. (2022) The role of m6A modification in pediatric cancer. *Biochimica et Biophysica Acta. Reviews on Cancer* 1877:188691.

[57] Cortini, M., Avnet, S., Baldini, N. (2017) Mesenchymal stroma: Role in osteosarcoma progression. *Cancer Letters* 405:90-99.

[58] Mirabello, L., Troisi, R. J., Savage, S. A. (2009) Osteosarcoma incidence and survival rates from 1973 to 2004: data from the Surveillance, Epidemiology, and End Results Program. *Cancer* 115:1531-1543.

[59] Mundy, G. R. (2002) Metastasis to bone: causes, consequences and therapeutic opportunities. *Nature Reviews. Cancer* 2:584-593.
[60] Chirgwin, J. M., Guise, T. A. (2000) Molecular mechanisms of tumor-bone interactions in osteolytic metastases. *Critical Reviews in Eukaryotic Gene Expression* 10:159-178.
[61] Moore, D. D., Luu, H. H. (2014) Osteosarcoma. *Cancer Treatment and Research* 162:65-92.
[62] Yadav, P., Subbarayalu, P., Medina, D., Nirzhor, S., Timilsina, S., Rajamanickam, S., Eedunuri, V. K., Gupta, Y., Zheng, S., Abdelfattah, N., Huang, Y., Vadlamudi, R., Hromas, R., Meltzer, P., Houghton, P., Chen, Y., Rao, M. K. (2022) M6A RNA Methylation Regulates Histone Ubiquitination to Support Cancer Growth and Progression. *Cancer Research* 82:1872-1889.
[63] Botter, S. M., Neri, D., Fuchs, B. (2014) Recent advances in osteosarcoma. *Current Opinion in Pharmacology* 16:15-23.
[64] Wang, Y., Zeng, L., Liang, C., Zan, R., Ji, W., Zhang, Z., Wei, Y., Tu, S., Dong, Y. (2019) Integrated analysis of transcriptome-wide m(6)A methylome of osteosarcoma stem cells enriched by chemotherapy. *Epigenomics* 11:1693-1715.
[65] Li, J., Rao, B., Yang, J., Liu, L., Huang, M., Liu, X., Cui, G., Li, C., Han, Q., Yang, H., Cui, X., Sun, R. (2020) Dysregulated m6A-Related Regulators Are Associated With Tumor Metastasis and Poor Prognosis in Osteosarcoma. *Frontiers in Oncology* 10:769.
[66] Miao, W., Chen, J., Jia, L., Ma, J., Song, D. (2019) The m6A methyltransferase METTL3 promotes osteosarcoma progression by regulating the m6A level of LEF1. *Biochem Biophys Res Commun* 516:719-725.
[67] Ling, Z., Chen, L., Zhao, J. (2020) m6A-dependent up-regulation of DRG1 by METTL3 and ELAVL1 promotes growth, migration, and colony formation in osteosarcoma. *Biosci Rep* 40.
[68] Zhou, L., Yang, C., Zhang, N., Zhang, X., Zhao, T., Yu, J. (2020) Silencing METTL3 inhibits the proliferation and invasion of osteosarcoma by regulating ATAD2. *Biomedicine & Pharmacotherapy,* 125:109964.
[69] Zhou, X., Yang, Y., Li, Y., Liang, G., Kang, D., Zhou, B., Li, Q. (2021) METTL3 Contributes to Osteosarcoma Progression by Increasing DANCR mRNA Stability via m6A Modification. *Frontiers in Cell and Developmental Biology* 9:784719.
[70] Zhang, C., Wan, J., Liu, Q., Long, F., Wen, Z., Liu, Y. (2022) METTL3 upregulates COPS5 expression in osteosarcoma in an m(6)A-related manner to promote osteosarcoma progression. *Experimental Cell Research* 420:113353.
[71] Meng, Y., Hao, D., Huang, Y., Jia, S., Zhang, J., He, X., Liu, D., Sun, L. (2021) Circular RNA circNRIP1 plays oncogenic roles in the progression of osteosarcoma. *Mammalian Genome: Official Journal of the International Mammalian Genome Society*.
[72] Wei, K., Gao, Y., Wang, B., Qu, Y. X. (2022) Methylation recognition protein YTH N6-methyladenosine RNA binding protein 1 (YTHDF1) regulates the proliferation, migration and invasion of osteosarcoma by regulating m6A level of CCR4-NOT transcription complex subunit 7 (CNOT7). *Bioengineered* 13:5236-5250.

[73] Wang, J., Wang, W., Huang, X., Cao, J., Hou, S., Ni, X., Peng, C., Liu, T. (2022) m6A-dependent upregulation of TRAF6 by METTL3 is associated with metastatic osteosarcoma. *Journal of Bone Oncology* 32:100411.

[74] Jiang, R., Dai, Z., Wu, J., Ji, S., Sun, Y., Yang, W. (2022) METTL3 stabilizes HDAC5 mRNA in an m(6)A-dependent manner to facilitate malignant proliferation of osteosarcoma cells. *Cell Death Discovery* 8:179.

[75] Li, H. B., Huang, G., Tu, J., Lv, D. M., Jin, Q. L., Chen, J. K., Zou, Y. T., Lee, D. F., Shen, J. N., Xie, X. B. (2022) METTL14-mediated epitranscriptome modification of MN1 mRNA promote tumorigenicity and all-trans-retinoic acid resistance in osteosarcoma. *EBioMedicine* 82:104142.

[76] Chen, S., Li, Y., Zhi, S., Ding, Z., Wang, W., Peng, Y., Huang, Y., Zheng, R., Yu, H., Wang, J., Hu, M., Miao, J., Li, J. (2020) WTAP promotes osteosarcoma tumorigenesis by repressing HMBOX1 expression in an m(6)A-dependent manner. *Cell Death Dis* 11:659.

[77] Ren, Z., Hu, Y., Sun, J., Kang, Y., Li, G., Zhao, H. (2022) N(6)-methyladenosine methyltransferase WTAP-stabilized FOXD2-AS1 promotes the osteosarcoma progression through m(6)A/FOXM1 axis. *Bioengineered* 13:7963-7973.

[78] Huang, H., Cui, X., Qin, X., Li, K., Yan, G., Lu, D., Zheng, M., Hu, Z., Lei, D., Lan, N., Zheng, L., Yuan, Z., Zhu, B., Zhao, J. (2022) Analysis and identification of m(6)A RNA methylation regulators in metastatic osteosarcoma. *Molecular Therapy. Nucleic Acids* 27:577-592.

[79] Yang, F., Liu, Y., Xiao, J., Li, B., Chen, Y., Hu, A., Zeng, J., Liu, Z., Liu, H. (2022) Circ-CTNNB1 drives aerobic glycolysis and osteosarcoma progression via m6A modification through interacting with RBM15. *Cell Proliferation*:e13344.

[80] Yuan, Y., Yan, G., He, M., Lei, H., Li, L., Wang, Y., He, X., Li, G., Wang, Q., Gao, Y., Qu, Z., Mei, Z., Shen, Z., Pu, J., Wang, A., Zhao, W., Jiang, H., Du, W., Yang, L. (2021) ALKBH5 suppresses tumor progression via an m(6)A-dependent epigenetic silencing of pre-miR-181b-1/YAP signaling axis in osteosarcoma. *Cell Death Dis* 12:60.

[81] Yang, Z., Cai, Z., Yang, C., Luo, Z., Bao, X. (2022) ALKBH5 regulates STAT3 activity to affect the proliferation and tumorigenicity of osteosarcoma via an m6A-YTHDF2-dependent manner. *EBioMedicine* 80:104019.

[82] Cao, D., Ge, S., Li, M. (2022) MiR-451a promotes cell growth, migration and EMT in osteosarcoma by regulating YTHDC1-mediated m6A methylation to activate the AKT/mTOR signaling pathway. *Journal of Bone Oncology* 33:100412.

[83] Liu, D., Li, Z., Zhang, K., Lu, D., Zhou, D., Meng, Y. (2022) N(6)-methyladenosine reader YTHDF3 contributes to the aerobic glycolysis of osteosarcoma through stabilizing PGK1 stability. *Journal of Cancer Research and Clinical Oncology*.

[84] Zhou, C., Zhang, Z., Zhu, X., Qian, G., Zhou, Y., Sun, Y., Yu, W., Wang, J., Lu, H., Lin, F., Shen, Z., Zheng, S. (2020) N6-Methyladenosine modification of TRIM7 positively regulates tumorigenesis and chemoresistance in osteosarcoma through ubiquitination of BRMS1. *EBioMedicine* 59:102955.

[85] Liu, Z., Liu, N., Huang, Z., Wang, W. (2020) METTL14 Overexpression Promotes Osteosarcoma Cell Apoptosis and Slows Tumor Progression via Caspase 3 Activation. *Cancer Manag Res* 12:12759-12767.

[86] Chen, S., Zhou, L., Wang, Y. (2020) ALKBH5-mediated m(6)A demethylation of lncRNA PVT1 plays an oncogenic role in osteosarcoma. *Cancer Cell Int* 20:34.

[87] Zeng, L., Chen, C., Yao, C. (2021) Histone Deacetylation Regulated by KDM1A to Suppress DACT1 in Proliferation and Migration of Cervical Cancer. *Analytical Cellular Pathology (Amsterdam)* 2021:5555452.

[88] Zhu, K., Jiang, B., Yang, Y., Hu, R., Liu, Z. (2017) DACT1 overexpression inhibits proliferation, enhances apoptosis, and increases daunorubicin chemosensitivity in KG-1α cells. *Tumor Biology : The Journal of the International Society for Oncodevelopmental Biology and Medicine* 39:1010428317711089.

[89] Lv, D., Ding, S., Zhong, L., Tu, J., Li, H., Yao, H., Zou, Y., Zeng, Z., Liao, Y., Wan, X., Wen, L., Xie, X. (2022) M(6)A demethylase FTO-mediated downregulation of DACT1 mRNA stability promotes Wnt signaling to facilitate osteosarcoma progression. *Oncogene* 41:1727-1741.

[90] Wu, Z. Y., Shi, Z. Y. (2022) The prognostic value and immune landscapes of m1A/m5C/m6A-associated lncRNA signature in osteosarcoma. *European Review for Medical and Pharmacological Sciences* 26:5868-5883.

[91] Wu, Z., Zhang, X., Chen, D., Li, Z., Wu, X., Wang, J., Deng, Y. (2021) N6-Methyladenosine-Related LncRNAs Are Potential Remodeling Indicators in the Tumor Microenvironment and Prognostic Markers in Osteosarcoma. *Frontiers in Immunology* 12:806189.

[92] Peng, S., Yi, Z., Liu, M. (2017) Ailanthone: a new potential drug for castration-resistant prostate cancer. *Chinese Journal of Cancer* 36:25.

[93] Ren, D., Yang, Q., Dai, Y., Guo, W., Du, H., Song, L., Peng, X. (2017) Oncogenic miR-210-3p promotes prostate cancer cell EMT and bone metastasis via NF-κB signaling pathway. *Molecular Cancer* 16:117.

[94] Li, E., Wei, B., Wang, X., Kang, R. (2020) METTL3 enhances cell adhesion through stabilizing integrin β1 mRNA via an m6A-HuR-dependent mechanism in prostatic carcinoma. *American Journal of Cancer Research* 10:1012-1025.

[95] Wen, S., Wei, Y., Zen, C., Xiong, W., Niu, Y., Zhao, Y. (2020) Long non-coding RNA NEAT1 promotes bone metastasis of prostate cancer through N6-methyladenosine. *Molecular Cancer* 19:171.

[96] Lang, C., Yin, C., Lin, K., Li, Y., Yang, Q., Wu, Z., Du, H., Ren, D., Dai, Y., Peng, X. (2021) m(6) A modification of lncRNA PCAT6 promotes bone metastasis in prostate cancer through IGF2BP2-mediated IGF1R mRNA stabilization. *Clinical and Translational Medicine* 11:e426.

[97] Zheng, Y., Gao, Y., Li, X., Si, S., Xu, H., Qi, F., Wang, J., Cheng, G., Hua, L., Yang, H. (2018) Long non-coding RNA NAP1L6 promotes tumor progression and predicts poor prognosis in prostate cancer by targeting Inhibin-β A. *OncoTargets and Therapy* 11:4965-4977.

[98] Zheng, Y., Qi, F., Li, L., Yu, B., Cheng, Y., Ge, M., Qin, C., Li, X. (2022) LncNAP1L6 activates MMP pathway by stabilizing the m6A-modified NAP1L2 to promote malignant progression in prostate cancer. *Cancer Gene Therapy*.

[99] Monteran, L., Ershaid, N., Sabah, I., Fahoum, I., Zait, Y., Shani, O., Cohen, N., Eldar-Boock, A., Satchi-Fainaro, R., Erez, N. (2020) Bone metastasis is associated with acquisition of mesenchymal phenotype and immune suppression in a model of spontaneous breast cancer metastasis. *Sci Rep* 10:13838.

[100] Jin, Y., Zhang, M., Duan, R., Yang, J., Yang, Y., Wang, J., Jiang, C., Yao, B., Li, L., Yuan, H., Zha, X., Ma, C. (2020) Long noncoding RNA FGF14-AS2 inhibits breast cancer metastasis by regulating the miR-370-3p/FGF14 axis. *Cell Death Discovery* 6:103.

[101] Zhang, M., Wang, J., Jin, Y., Zheng, Q., Xing, M., Tang, Y., Ma, Y., Li, L., Yao, B., Wu, H., Ma, C. (2022) YTHDF2-mediated FGF14-AS2 decay promotes osteolytic metastasis of breast cancer by enhancing RUNX2 mRNA translation. *British Journal of cancer*.

[102] Macedo, F., Ladeira, K., Pinho, F., Saraiva, N., Bonito, N., Pinto, L., Goncalves, F. (2017) Bone Metastases: An Overview. *Oncology Reviews* 11:321.

[103] Coleman, R. E., Croucher, P. I., Padhani, A. R., Clézardin, P., Chow, E., Fallon, M., Guise, T., Colangeli, S., Capanna, R., Costa, L. (2020) Bone metastases. *Nature Reviews. Disease Primers* 6:83.

Chapter 2

The "Communicator" Role of Extracellular Vesicles in Bone Metastasis

Zicai Dong[1]
and Yueqi Chen[2,*]

[1] Department of Biomedical Materials Science,
Third Military Medical University (Army Medical University),
Chongqing, People's Republic of China
[2] Department of Orthopedics, Southwest Hospital,
Third Military Medical University (Army Medical University),
Chongqing, People's Republic of China

Abstract

Cancer-associated bone metastasis acts as the critical poor progression for the malignant tumors, which may be involved in the procedure of bone remodeling including osteoclasts-mediated bone resorption and osteoblasts-mediated bone regeneration. Several crucial cytokines secreted among osteoclasts and osteoblasts could make close interaction to promote cell differentiation, maturation and perform functions. In addition, many cell factors such as transforming growth factor beta (TGF-β), fibroblast growth factor (FGF), insulin growth factor (IGF), platelet-derived growth factor (PDGF), and bone morphogenetic proteins (BMPs) from the bone matrix during bone resorption lesions could induce the differentiation of MSCs into osteoblasts. In turn, osteoblasts might participate in osteoclastogenesis through secreting M-CSF and RANKL. Tumor associated bone metastasis exhibits osteolytic and osteogenic lesions. Extracellular vesicles could make coupling effects on

---

[*] Corresponding Author's Email: chenyueqi1012@sina.com.

In: New Research on Bone Metastasis
Editor: Joseph Gerfried
ISBN: 979-8-88697-799-8
© 2023 Nova Science Publishers, Inc.

bone remodeling process through their complex vesicular contents such as non-coding RNA, protein and so on.

In this chapter, we have summarized the role of extracellular vesicles in the procedure of bone metastasis during the micro-environment. In detail, it is well illustrated how breast cancer cell-derived extracellular vesicles affect the proliferation, differentiation and functions of osteoblasts and osteoclasts. In addition, it is also noted that the extracellular vesicles modulate the distant metastasis procedure of multiple myeloma and osteosarcoma from the original site to bone tissue. Elaborating on the role of extracellular vesicles in tumor associated bone metastasis may provide novel insight for the treatment of tumor bone metastasis.

Introduction

As a class of small membranous vesicles, extracellular vesicles (EVs) are derived from cells and move into the extracellular matrix, involved in processes such as cell communication, cell migration, angiogenesis, and tumor metastasis. EVs are widely present in various body fluids and cell supernatants, which stably carry several important signaling molecules [1, 2]. EVs are often classified in accordance with their morphology, contents, generation mode, and mechanism of release [3]. The current common classification is mainly based on vesicle diameter: approximately 100 nm diameter of vesicles are defined as exosomes, approximately 1 um as microvesicles (MVs), and greater than 1um as apoptotic bodies [4, 5]. Another classification method is similar to the above one: vesicles are classified into three groups including small, medium, and large vesicles with diameters <100 nm, <200 nm, and >200 nm [6]. Different sizes of extracellular vesicles have different contents and compositions and perform different biological functions. Due to the overlap in size, density, contents, membrane orientation and surface molecules of the various subtypes of vesicles, existing methods of EVs isolation and analysis are difficult to achieve effective discrimination. There is no unified standard nomenclature, so in this paper, exosomes, MVs, extranuclear granules and particles are collectively referred to as EVs.

EVs are released from different cells with different contents, act as messengers for different biological signals and perform a variety of biological functions among cells. Back in 1996, researchers found that exosomes from human and murine B lymphocytes restricted the T cell immune response by inducing antigen-specific MHC class II [7]. Since then, the study of EVs in the immune response has been kicked off. EVs-induced transport mechanisms involving cell-environment interactions and cell-cell communications have not yet been fully revealed. Metastasis is a critical stage in the development of tumors which poses significant challenges in treatment process. EVs mediate cell-cell communications among tumor cells and the interactions with the micro-environment of distant organs, performing important functions in pre-metastatic niche (PMN) formations and metastasis [8]. Various procedures of metastasis depend on tumor exosome-mediated cancer organ tropism [9]. Bone is the third most preferred organ for cancer metastasis, which is next to lung and liver. Bone metastasis could lead to a series of serious complications including skeleton ache, hypercalcemia, brittle bones, and pathological fractures, which are referred to as skeletal-related events (SREs)[10, 11].

In conclusion, EVs play irreplaceable and significant roles in the bone microenvironment and cancer bone tropism. Exploring the biological functions of EVs and understanding the mechanisms that govern the metastasis process by EVs may provide new ideas for the treatment of bone metastases.

Bone Remodeling and Bone Metastasis

Osteoblasts (OB) are mainly derived from mesenchymal progenitor cells in the stroma of the inner and outer periosteum and bone marrow, and specifically secrete a variety of bioactive substances that regulate and make effects on the process of bone formation and resorption. At different stages of maturation, osteoblasts are expressed *in vivo* in four different forms: pre-osteoblast, osteoblast, osteocyte and bones lining cell. Osteoblasts perform crucial functions in the process of bone formation, which are involved in bone matrix synthesis and secretion, as well as mineralization.

Osteoclasts (OC) are the main functional cells in bone resorption and play an essential role in bone development, growth, repair and reconstruction. Osteoclasts are a special type of terminally differentiated cell that originated from the hematopoietic monocyte-macrophage system and can be formed into giant multinucleated cells by the fusion of their mononuclear precursor cells. In contrast to osteoblasts, which are responsible for new bone formation, osteoclasts are responsible for bone breakdown and resorption. Specifically, osteoclasts adhere to the area of old bone, secret acid to dissolve the mineral and protease to digest the bone matrix respectively, forming a bone resorption trap. Subsequently, osteoblasts migrate to the resorbed area and mineralize and form new bone by secreting the bone matrix. The balance between osteoclastic and osteogenic processes is essential to maintain normal dynamic balance of bone mass.

Bone remodeling is an exquisite balance of these osteoclastic and osteoblastic activities. Osteoblasts and osteoclasts are closely linked to each other by EVs containing proteins and non-coding RNAs. Macrophage colony-stimulating factor (M-CSF), nuclear factor kappa-B ligand receptor activator (RANKL) and the RANKL receptor decoy osteoprotegerin (OPG), secreted by osteoblasts, activate the proliferation of osteoclasts. During osteoclast bone resorption, transforming growth factor beta (TGF-β), fibroblast growth factor (FGF), insulin growth factor (IGF), platelet-derived lineage factor (PDGF), bone morphogenetic proteins (BMPs), and sphingosine-1-phosphate (S1P) are released from the bone matrix. These factors could promote the osteogenic differentiation of MSCs [12]. In conclusion, these proteins released by OBs and OCs participate in the procedures of the proliferation, differentiation, and maturation of OBs and OCs. Intercellular communication between OBs and OCs forms a beneficial cycle through EV cargoes.

Bone metastasis exhibit osteolytic and osteogenic lesions, which severely damages the beneficial balance of bone remodeling. Elucidating the mechanisms of EV involvement in bone metastasis might be helpful for exploring therapeutic strategy of bone metastasis. Bone metastasis is a cascade of complex processes such as tumor cells migrate and invade into the bone specifically, and subsequently acquire bone-like characteristics to invade the bone marrow. Eventually, there are communications between the tumor cells and the normal constituent cells of the bone. It disrupts the normal physiological metabolic processes of bone and creates suitable microenvironment for tumor proliferation and invasion [13]. The role of EVs in these processes has been widely reported. The specific components of EVs related to bone metastases depends on the specific primary tumor type.

Bone Metastasis and EVs

Prostate cancer, breast cancer and lung cancer are top 3 most frequent primary tumors of bone metastasis. In patients with prostate and breast cancer, approximately 70% are accompanied by bone metastasis. Lung cancer patients have a lower rate of skeletal metastases, about 30-40%.

Prostate Cancer

Prostate cancer (PCa) is one of the cancers that exhibits cancer metastasis tropism to the bone in men, however, the specific mechanisms of bone metastasis in PCa is not fully illustrated. More and more researchers focus on the EVs derived from PCa to reveal the interactions of cancer cell with bone. PCa-related bone metastasis exhibits both osteogenic and osteolytic lesions. There is a coupling role between these two kinds of lesions, in which bone resorption plays an essential role in subsequent bone formation in the early phase of PCa invasion in bone. Researchers found that PC3 cells, a type of human PCa cells, stimulated osteoclastogenesis in RAW 264.7 cells and the proliferation of human osteoblasts by secreting related EVs [14].

On the contrary, TRAMP-C1 cells, as a murine PCa line, decreases the expression of tartrate-resistant acid phosphatase (TRAP), matrix metallopeptidase (MMP)-9, cathepsin K (CTSK), and so on, which are established as markers of OCs fusion and differentiation, thereby inhibiting OC lineage development [15]. In addition, metastatic PCa cell line MDA PCa 2b secreted EVs containing miR-141-3p have been proved to promote OB development and increased OPG expression, an osteoclast inhibitory factor [16]. Hsa-miR-940 enriched-EVs, released by PCa cells, also promoted osteogenic differentiation of human MSCs [17]. On the other hand, RNAs contained-EVs deliver a set of PCa-RNAs to osteoblast, which means that RNA component of EV cargoes contributed to bone metastasis [18]. Interestingly, osteoblasts contribute to the proliferation of PC3 cells by secreting EVs containing specific proteins that function in the mineralization stage [19].

Breast Cancer

In the progression of breast cancer (BCa), the patients have a sky-high rate of bone metastasis, approximately 70%. BCa bone metastasis mainly exhibits osteolytic lesions. BCa-derived EVs contributed to establishing a premetastatic niche by inhibiting the proliferation of CD8 and CD4 T-cell NK cytotoxic activity. It is favorable for BCa to escape immune surveillance and promote metastasis [20]. BCa-derived EVs containing miR-218 directly downregulates type I collagen in osteoblasts and subsequently repress osteoblast differentiation. It is a result of increased cancer secretion of inhibin β subunits and elevated Timp3 expression in osteoblasts [21]. BCa secreted L-plastin and PRDX4 mediate osteoclast activation through stimulation of calcium oscillations and nuclear translocation of nuclear factor of activated T cells (NFAT) c1 transcription factor [22]. MiR-222/223 containing-EVs, which is released by bone marrow-mesenchymal stem cells (BM-MSCs), promote quiescence in a subset of cancer cells and lead to drug resistance [23].

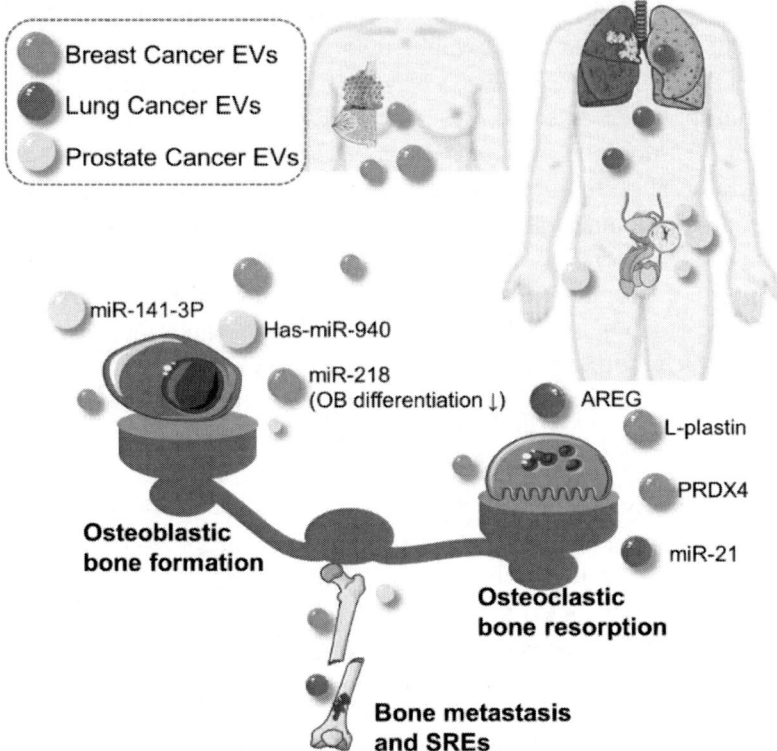

Figure 1. EVs mediated cell-cell communications among tumor cells and the interactions with the micro-environment of distant organs. EVs, derived from primary cancer, contain various proteins and nuclear acids, promote the pre-metastatic niche (PMN) formations and disrupt bone remodeling through the interruption of osteoblastogenesis and osteoclastogenesis. It turns out bone metastasis and skeletal-related events (SREs).

Lung Cancer

The bone metastasis of lung cancer (LCa) is apt to exhibit osteolytic lesions due to the EVs derived from LCa mainly stimulate osteoclastogenesis. Human non-small cell lung cancer (NSCLC) disrupted the RANKL/RANK/OPG system, which plays a pivotal role in bone remodeling by regulating osteoclast formation and activity [24]. NSCLC-EVs containing Amphiregulin (AREG) induced osteoclast differentiation through the activation of EGFR pathway and subsequently increased expression of RANKL in pre-osteoclasts [25]. Moreover, lung adenocarcinoma cell-derived miR-21-EVs transferred from lung adenocarcinoma cells to osteoclast progenitor cells to facilitates osteoclastogenesis [26].

Perspectives on EV Applications

There is no currently sufficient evidence for the clinical applications of EVs in cancer therapy. However, as the important roles of EVs in tumorigenesis and cancer metastasis continue to be revealed, new ideas for EVs-based tumor therapy are being explored. At present, the researches of cancer therapy based on EVs focus on these three aspects: the application of EVs as biomarkers in the diagnosis and prognosis of disease, as the vehicle of drug delivery system (DDS) and vaccination, and EV-targeting therapeutic application.

EV Components as Diagnostic or Prognostic Biomarkers

A biopsy is an effective method that is required in the definitive diagnosis of most cancers, however, traditional tissue biopsies cause a great deal of pain to the patient and result in many side effects such as the spread and metastasis of the cancer. EV-based liquid biopsy may achieve predictive diagnosis and treatment, through many body fluid specimens, such as blood, saliva, or semen. As we mentioned before, EVs are lipid membranous vesicles and encapsulate specific proteins and nuclear acids from original cells.

There are many advantages of EV-based liquid biopsy compared with conventional tissue biopsy. The miRNAs and proteins in EVs are widely explored and expected to serve as new biomarkers of cancers. The biomarkers on the surface and content of EVs may represent the true status of diseases. Messenger RNA (mRNA), as another component of EVs, serves biomarkers for cancers as well [27]. A configurable microwell-patterned micro-fluidic digital bioassay chip has been developed to assess the mRNA level in EVs. Indeed, the absolute quantification of mRNAs in tumor derived EVs exhibits high sensitivity and specificity [28]. Moreover, EV-based liquid biopsy is much more convenient and easier to collect than conventional tissue biopsy because of abundance of EVs in body fluid such as blood, saliva, and semen. However, EV testing is still time-consuming and must meet several additional criteria, including high cost, high sensitivity, high specificity, and relevance to the clinical course of the disease [29].

Recently, ExoScreen, a new and ultrasensitive EV detection method based on the combination of antibody against EV specific marker, could detect EVs in a small volume of body fluids or conditioned medium without sample purification [30]. It offered the possibility for EV detection in clinical samples with low degree of purity. Furthermore, the ExoScreen assay was applied by Yoshioka et al. to detect EVs with CD147, an early-stage colorectal cancer biomarker, and CD9 double-positive in early colorectal cancer samples with invasion of the submucosa [30]. More applications of EVs in cancer diagnosis have been reported. PRINS, a long noncoding RNA, shows high expression in multiple myeloma (MM) patients and monoclonal gammopathy of undetermined significance (MGUS) patients, which might serve invasive marker of both MM and MGUS. PRINS expression in circulating EVs from peripheral blood serum helped diagnose MM and MGUS [31]. So far, there is a lack of adequate clinical application of EVs in cancer diagnosis and prognosis, but a growing number of studies indicate promising prospects.

EVs as the Vehicle of Drug Delivery Systems (DDS) and Vaccinations

The use of anticancer drugs remains the mainstay of cancer treatment, both in patients after tumor resection and in patients with progressive cancer whose tumors cannot be removed. However, it is difficult for drugs to accumulate at the tumor site, which fails to avoid the effects on surrounding normal cells. Anti-cancer drug therapy suffers from high side effects and low drug concentrations at the tumor site. It is a promising new research field that uses EVs as DDS agents in recent years. EVs could bind to specific receptors through specific membrane proteins and lipids, which may serve as effective drug-delivery tools.

On the other hand, it is generally difficult to filter and expel EVs in the kidney. Conversely, EVs in tumor and inflammatory tissues show tendency to flow out of the blood vessels and accumulate in the tissue. It is known as enhanced permeation and retention (EPR) effect [32]. A doxorubicin (DXR) encapsulated EV delivery system with engineering the immature dendritic cells (imDCs) has been used for targeted tumor therapy. To increase interactions with αv-expressing target cells, engineered imDCs express the EV membrane protein Lamp2b fused to αv integrin-specific iRGD peptide (CRGDKGPDC) [33]. iRGD DXR-EVs effectively suppressed tumor cell in murine breast cancer, with high efficiency and low toxicity compared to free doxorubicin. It suggested that EVs modified by targeting ligands can be used as the vehicle of DDS with great potential value for clinical applications. Moreover, Ohno et al. achieved targeting by modifying donor cells to express a transmembrane structural domain platelet-derived growth factor receptor fused to the GE11 peptide. EVs efficiently delivered miRNA to breast cancer cells that express epidermal growth factor receptor (EGFR) [34].

In addition to DDS, EVs also serve as vehicles in vaccination. Dendritic cells (DCs), professional antigen presenting cells, secrete antigen presenting EVs, which express functional Major Histocompatibility Complex (MHC) class I and class II, and T-cell costimulatory molecules. Tumor peptide-pulsed DC-derived EVs activated specific cytotoxic T lymphocytes. Exosome-based cell-free vaccines suppressed murine tumor growth [35]. Regrettably, there is no report on applicable method to accumulate and store EVs as DDS vehicle in the bone. The development of bone-related EVs as DDS to skeletal system researches are challenging but desiderative.

Strategies of EV-Targeting Therapy

As we mentioned before, EVs mediated cell-cell communications among tumor cells and the interactions with the micro-environment of distant organs during tumor progression. Therefore, EVs from cancer cells might be effective therapeutic targets. Reduction of cancer-derived EV cargo transmission may inhibit metastasis in tumors. Primarily, several studies described the inhibition of EV production suppressed cancer progression. Ceramide, synthesized by neutral sphingomyelinase (nSMase) 2, triggers budding of EVs into multivesicular endosomes. Knockdown of nSMase2 or addition of its inhibitor GW4869 resulted in inhibition of angiogenesis and metastasis in a xenograft mouse model by the reduction of EV secretion and miR-210 transcription [36, 37]. Lysosome-associated membrane protein (LAMP) 2, an endocytic receptor on human monocyte-derived dendritic cells (MoDC), is related to endocytosis. Knockdown of LAMP-2 inhibited the production of highly immunogenic EV, induced robust proliferation of CD4 cells and improved the therapeutic effect of sunitinib in pancreatic neuroendocrine tumors [38].

Eliminating circulating EVs might be another therapeutic strategy in cancer patients. Researchers revealed that treatment with cancer-specific antigens, such as human-specific anti-CD9 or anti-CD63 antibodies, significantly eliminated antibody-tagged cancer-derived EVs through macrophages, which decreased breast cancer metastasis to the lungs, lymph nodes, and thoracic cavity [39]. However, CD9 and CD63 are not specific markers of cancer-derived EV. Further studies on eliminating EVs using a cancer-specific antigen need to be conducted. Human epidermal growth factor receptor type 2 (HER2) is breast cancer-specific EV surface protein. Marleau et al. developed the hemofiltration system, an exosome extracorporeal hemofiltration system that depends on an affinity plasmapheresis platform, which could specifically capture circulating HER2-positive EVs [40].

Disruption of the absorption of EVs might be another potential therapeutic strategy. However, there is no efficient application on cancer bone metastasis therapy as we know. EVs are taken up by a variety of endocytic pathways, such as clathrin-dependent endocytosis, caveolin-mediated uptake, phagocytosis, micropinocytosis and lipid raft-mediated fusion of the plasma and endosomal membranes [41]. Targeting the specific molecules involved in the reception of cell-cell communication could be potential strategy to disrupt the resorption of EV with high specificity.

Conclusion

Cancer has always been a disease that seriously affects the quality of patient's life, especially in an ageing society where cancer incidence and mortality rates are increasing. The current application of anti-cancer drugs based on the resection of solid tumors has important clinical efficacy. However, the targeting and specificity of drugs, and how to maintain effective concentrations of anti-cancer drugs at the tumor site are challenging in cancer treatment.

EVs, widely present in various body fluids and cell supernatants, participate in many biologic processes such as cell communication, cell migration, angiogenesis and tumor cell growth. EVs stably carry a number of important signaling molecules. The studies of EV-related functions have become research hotspots and are expected to play a role in the early diagnosis of many diseases. We presented the important role of EVs in bone remodeling and tumor related bone metastasis. Research advances in EVs-related tumor treatment strategies are summarized. It is believed that EVs detection possesses important research value in tumor diagnosis and prognosis, DDS and vaccine vehicles, and EV-targeted therapy.

EVs as a biomarker lend themselves to their characteristic of encapsulating multiple molecules that are specific to the type of cancer, and EV-based liquid biopsies offer many advantages. Liquid biopsies are more readily available than traditional tissue biopsies. In addition, these molecules exhibit high cancer specificity, which may be unique therapeutic targets of drugs against cancers. EVs are also a possible drug delivery vehicle that can efficiently carry a variety of bioactive drugs and deliver them to cancer cells. Despite the remarkable progress in the purification methods of EVs, there are still many problems with current studies s before future clinical applications. Therefore, elucidating the precise mechanisms of the EV uptake pathway is required for more efficient delivery. The discovery of tumor-specific EV secretion pathways and/or proteins could significantly improve EV-targeted therapies.

References

[1] Jiang, C., Zhang, N., Hu, X. & Wang, H. Tumor-associated exosomes promote lung cancer metastasis through multiple mechanisms. *Mol. Cancer* 20, 117 (2021).

[2] Dai, J., Su, Y., Zhong, S., Cong, L., Liu, B., Yang, J., Tao, Y., He, Z., Chen, C., & Jiang, Y. Exosomes: key players in cancer and potential therapeutic strategy. *Signal Transduct. Target. Ther.* 5, 145 (2020).

[3] van der Pol, E., Böing, A. N., Harrison, P., Sturk, A. & Nieuwland, R. Classification, functions, and clinical relevance of extracellular vesicles. *Pharmacol. Rev.* 64, 676–705 (2012).

[4] Thietart, Sara, and Pierre-Emmanuel Rautou. Extracellular vesicles as biomarkers in liver diseases: A clinician's point of view. *J. Hepatol.* 73, (2020).

[5] van Niel, G., D'Angelo, G. & Raposo, G. Shedding light on the cell biology of extracellular vesicles. *Nat. Rev. Mol. Cell Biol.* 19, 213–228 (2018).

[6] Théry, C., Witwer, K. W., Aikawa, E., Alcaraz, M. J., Anderson, J. D., Andriantsitohaina, R. et al. Minimal information for studies of extracellular vesicles 2018 (MISEV2018): a position statement of the International Society for Extracellular Vesicles and update of the MISEV2014 guidelines. *J. Extracell. Vesicles* 7, 1535750 (2018).

[7] Raposo, G., Nijman H. W., Stoorvogel W., Liejendekker R., Harding C. V., Melief C. J., and Geuze H. J. B lymphocytes secrete antigen-presenting vesicles. *J. Exp. Med.* 183, 1161–1172 (1996).

[8] Wortzel, I., Dror, S., Kenific, C. M. & Lyden, D. Exosome-Mediated Metastasis: Communication from a Distance. *Dev. Cell* 49, 347–360 (2019).

[9] Hoshino, A., Costa-Silva, B., Shen, T.-L., Rodrigues, G., Hashimoto, A., Tesic Mark, et al. Tumor exosome integrins determine organotropic metastasis. *Nature* 527, 329–335 (2015).

[10] Yang, M., Liu, C. & Yu, X. Skeletal-related adverse events during bone metastasis of breast cancer: current status. *Discov. Med.* 27, 211–220 (2019).

[11] Coleman, R. E. Clinical Features of Metastatic Bone Disease and Risk of Skeletal Morbidity. *Clin. Cancer Res.* 12, 6243s–6249s (2006).

[12] Kim, J.-M., Lin, C., Stavre, Z., Greenblatt, M. B. & Shim, J.-H. Osteoblast-Osteoclast Communication and Bone Homeostasis. *Cells* 9, 2073 (2020).

[13] Tamura, T., Yoshioka, Y., Sakamoto, S., Ichikawa, T. & Ochiya, T. Extracellular Vesicles in Bone Metastasis: Key Players in the Tumor Microenvironment and Promising Therapeutic Targets. *Int. J. Mol. Sci.* 21, 6680 (2020).

[14] Inder, K. L., Ruelcke J. E., Petelin L., Moon H., Choi E., Rae J., Blumenthal A., Hutmacher D., Saunders N. A., Stow J. L., Parton R. G., Hill M. M.. Cavin-1/PTRF alters prostate cancer cell-derived extracellular vesicle content and internalization to attenuate extracellular vesicle-mediated osteoclastogenesis and osteoblast proliferation. *J. Extracell. Vesicles* 3, (2014).

[15] Karlsson, T., Lundholm, M., Widmark, A. & Persson, E. Tumor Cell-Derived Exosomes from the Prostate Cancer Cell Line TRAMP-C1 Impair Osteoclast Formation and Differentiation. *PloS One* 11, e0166284 (2016).

[16] Ye, Y., Ye, Y., Li, S.-L., Ma, Y.-Y., Diao, Y.-J., Yang, L., Su, M.-Q., Li, Z., Ji, Y., Wang, J., Lei, L., Fan, W.-X., Li, L.-X., Xu, Y., & Hao, X.-K. Exosomal miR-141-3p regulates osteoblast activity to promote the osteoblastic metastasis of prostate cancer. *Oncotarget* 8, 94834–94849 (2017).

[17] Hashimoto, K., Ochi, H., Sunamura, S., Kosaka, N., Mabuchi, Y., Fukuda, T., Yao, K., Kanda, H., Ae, K, Okawa, A., Akazawa, C., Ochiya, T., Futakuchi, M., Takeda, S., Sato, S. Cancer-secreted hsa-miR-940 induces an osteoblastic phenotype in the bone metastatic microenvironment via targeting ARHGAP1 and FAM134A. *Proc. Natl. Acad. Sci. U. S. A.* 115, 2204–2209 (2018).

[18] Probert, C., Dottorini T., Speakman A., Hunt S., Nafee T., Fazeli A., Wood S., Brown J. E., James V. Communication of prostate cancer cells with bone cells via extracellular vesicle RNA; a potential mechanism of metastasis. *Oncogene* 38, 1751–1763 (2019).

[19] Morhayim, J., van de Peppel J., Demmers J. A. A., Kocer G., Nigg A. L., van Driel M., Chiba H., van Leeuwen J. P. Proteomic signatures of extracellular vesicles secreted by nonmineralizing and mineralizing human osteoblasts and stimulation of tumor cell growth. *FASEB J. Off. Publ. Fed. Am. Soc. Exp. Biol.* 29, 274–285 (2015).

[20] Wen, S. W., Sceneay, J., Lima, L. G., Wong, C. S. F., Becker, M., Krumeich, S., Lobb, R. J., Castillo, V., Wong, K. N., Ellis, S., Parker, B. S., & Möller, A. The Biodistribution and Immune Suppressive Effects of Breast Cancer-Derived Exosomes. *Cancer Res.* 76, 6816–6827 (2016).

[21] Liu, X., Cao M., Palomares M., Wu X., Li A., Yan W., Fong M. Y., Chan W-C, Wang S. E. Metastatic breast cancer cells overexpress and secrete miR-218 to regulate type I collagen deposition by osteoblasts. *Breast Cancer Res. BCR* 20, 127 (2018).

[22] Tiedemann, K., Sadvakassova, G., Mikolajewicz, N., Juhas, M., Sabirova, Z., Tabariès, S., Gettemans, J., Siegel, P. M., & Komarova, S. V. Exosomal Release of L-Plastin by Breast Cancer Cells Facilitates Metastatic Bone Osteolysis. *Transl. Oncol.* 12, 462–474 (2019).

[23] Bliss, S. A., Sinha, G., Sandiford, O. A., Williams, L. M., Engelberth, D. J., Guiro, K., Isenalumhe, L. L., Greco, S. J., Ayer, S., Bryan, M., Kumar, R., Ponzio, N. M., Rameshwar, P. Mesenchymal Stem Cell-Derived Exosomes Stimulate Cycling Quiescence and Early Breast Cancer Dormancy in Bone Marrow. *Cancer Res.* 76, 5832–5844 (2016).

[24] Peng, X., Guo, W., Ren, T., Lou, Z., Lu, X., Zhang, S., Lu, Q., Sun, Y. Differential expression of the RANKL/RANK/OPG system is associated with bone metastasis in human non-small cell lung cancer. *PloS One* 8, e58361 (2013).

[25] Taverna, S., Taverna, S., Pucci, M., Giallombardo, M., Di Bella, M. A., Santarpia, M., Reclusa, P., Gil-Bazo, I., Rolfo, C., & Alessandro, R. Amphiregulin contained in NSCLC-exosomes induces osteoclast differentiation through the activation of EGFR pathway. *Sci. Rep.* 7, 3170 (2017).

[26] Xu, Z., Liu, X., Wang, H., Li, J., Dai, L., Li, J., & Dong, C. Lung adenocarcinoma cell-derived exosomal miR-21 facilitates osteoclastogenesis. *Gene* 666, 116–122 (2018).

[27] Yokoi, A., Yokoi, A., Yoshioka, Y., Yamamoto, Y., Ishikawa, M., Ikeda, S., Kato, T., Kiyono, T., Takeshita, F., Kajiyama, H., Kikkawa, F., & Ochiya, T. Malignant extracellular vesicles carrying MMP1 mRNA facilitate peritoneal dissemination in ovarian cancer. *Nat. Commun.* 8, 14470 (2017).

[28] Zhang, P., Crow, J., Lella, D., Zhou, X., Samuel, G., Godwin, A. K., & Zeng, Y. Ultrasensitive quantification of tumor mRNAs in extracellular vesicles with an integrated microfluidic digital analysis chip. *Lab. Chip* 18, 3790–3801 (2018).

[29] Yamamoto, T., Kosaka, N. & Ochiya, T. Latest advances in extracellular vesicles: from bench to bedside. *Sci. Technol. Adv. Mater.* 20, 746–757 (2019).

[30] Yoshioka, Y., Kosaka, N., Konishi, Y., Ohta, H., Okamoto, H., Sonoda, H., Nonaka, R., Yamamoto, H., Ishii, H., Mori, M., Furuta, K., Nakajima, T., Hayashi, H., Sugisaki, H., Higashimoto, H., Kato, T., Takeshita, F., & Ochiya, T. Ultra-sensitive liquid biopsy of circulating extracellular vesicles using ExoScreen. *Nat. Commun.* 5, 3591 (2014).

[31] Sedlarikova, L., Bollova, B., Radova, L., Brozova, L., Jarkovsky, J., Almasi, M., Penka, M., Kuglík, P., Sandecká, V., Stork, M., Pour, L., & Sevcikova, S. Circulating exosomal long noncoding RNA PRINS-First findings in monoclonal gammopathies. *Hematol. Oncol.* 36, (2018).

[32] Sun, D., Zhuang, X., Zhang, S., Deng, Z.-B., Grizzle, W., Miller, D., & Zhang, H.-G. Exosomes are endogenous nanoparticles that can deliver biological information between cells. *Adv. Drug Deliv. Rev.* 65, 342–347 (2013).

[33] Tian, Y., Li, S., Song, J., Ji, T., Zhu, M., Anderson, G. J., Wei, J., & Nie, G.. A doxorubicin delivery platform using engineered natural membrane vesicle exosomes for targeted tumor therapy. *Biomaterials* 35, 2383–2390 (2014).

[34] Ohno, S., Takanashi, M., Sudo, K., Ueda, S., Ishikawa, A., Matsuyama, N., Fujita, K., Mizutani, T., Ohgi, T., Ochiya, T., Gotoh, N., Kuroda, M. Systemically injected

exosomes targeted to EGFR deliver antitumor microRNA to breast cancer cells. *Mol. Ther. J. Am. Soc. Gene Ther.* 21, (2013).

[35] Zitvogel, L., Regnault, A., Lozier, A., Wolfers, J., Flament, C., Tenza, D., Ricciardi-Castagnoli, P., Raposo, G., & Amigorena, S. Eradication of established murine tumors using a novel cell-free vaccine: dendritic cell-derived exosomes. *Nat. Med.* 4, 594–600 (1998).

[36] Trajkovic, K., Hsu, C., Chiantia, S., Rajendran, L., Wenzel, D., Wieland, F., Schwille, P., Brügger, B., & Simons, M. Ceramide triggers budding of exosome vesicles into multivesicular endosomes. *Science* 319, 1244–1247 (2008).

[37] Kosaka, N., Iguchi, H., Hagiwara, K., Yoshioka, Y., Takeshita, F., & Ochiya, T. Neutral sphingomyelinase 2 (nSMase2)-dependent exosomal transfer of angiogenic microRNAs regulate cancer cell metastasis. *J. Biol. Chem.* 288, (2013).

[38] Leone, D. A., Peschel, A., Brown, M., Schachner, H., Ball, M. J., Gyuraszova, M., Salzer-Muhar, U., Fukuda, M., Vizzardelli, C., Bohle, B., Rees, A. J., Kain R. Surface LAMP-2 Is an Endocytic Receptor That Diverts Antigen Internalized by Human Dendritic Cells into Highly Immunogenic Exosomes. *J. Immunol. Baltim. Md 1950* 199, 531–546 (2017).

[39] Nishida-Aoki, N., Tominaga, N., Takeshita, F., Sonoda, H., Yoshioka, Y., Ochiya, T. Disruption of Circulating Extracellular Vesicles as a Novel Therapeutic Strategy against Cancer Metastasis. *Mol. Ther. J. Am. Soc. Gene Ther.* 25, 181–191 (2017).

[40] Marleau, A. M., Chen, C.-S., Joyce, J. A. & Tullis, R. H. Exosome removal as a therapeutic adjuvant in cancer. *J. Transl. Med.* 10, 134 (2012).

[41] Mulcahy, L. A., Pink, R. C. & Carter, D. R. F. Routes and mechanisms of extracellular vesicle uptake. *J. Extracell. Vesicles* 3, (2014).

Chapter 3

Metastatic Disease of the Spine

Balaji Zacharia[*]
Department of Orthopedics,
Government Medical College, Manjeri, Kerala, India

Abstract

The spine is the most common site of skeletal metastasis. The breast, prostate, lung, thyroid, and kidney are tumors metastasizing to the spine. Hematogenous spread through the Batson plexus is the most typical mode of spread. Back pain is a common symptom. Spine metastasis also leads to vertebral compression fractures, deformity, and neurological deficits. Radiologically, there are osteolytic, osteosclerotic, and mixed types. Some metastases are radiosensitive, and others are radioresistant. Routine blood investigations, serum calcium, phosphorus, alkaline phosphatase, radiographs of the spine and chest, contrast-enhanced CT scans of the abdomen and chest, bone scans, and PET scans are common investigations. Primary tumor, epidural compression, type of lesion, stability of the segment, and general health of the patient influence the treatment. Treatment is a multimodal approach. Radiotherapy, stereotactic surgery, surgery combined with radiotherapy, and decompressive surgery are various modalities of treatment.

In this chapter, we describe the etiology, pathogenesis, presentations, investigations, classifications, and management of spinal metastasis.

Keywords: spine metastasis, metastatic disease of the spine, radiotherapy, SBRT, separation surgery

---

[*] Corresponding Author's Email: balaji.zacharia@gmail.com.

In: New Research on Bone Metastasis
Editor: Joseph Gerfried
ISBN: 979-8-88697-799-8
© 2023 Nova Science Publishers, Inc.

Introduction

Metastatic bone disease is on the rise. Advanced technologies for the detection of metastasis and its management are the reason for the increased incidence. The annual incidence of spinal metastatic diseases (SMDs) is 10 to 30% of all diagnosed cancers [1]. The spine is the most common site of skeletal metastasis. Approximately 40 to 70% of terminal cancer patients have spine metastasis. Patients between 40 and 65 years are commonly affected. A total of 9.6% of patients develop epidural compression [2]. The size and distribution of marrow are the determining factors for the site of occurrence. The lumbar vertebrae are the most common site, followed by the dorsal and cervical vertebrae. Due to the smaller dorsal spinal canal, the thoracic spine is the most common site of symptomatic spinal metastasis. Multiple myeloma is the most typical tumor metastasizing to the spine [3]. SMD can affect the functions of the spine, such as ambulation, maintaining an erect posture, and protecting the spinal cord and nerve roots.

The vertebral body is the most common site of involvement. Pedicle destruction is the earliest radiographic sign. CT scans in such cases show both pedicle and vertebral body destruction [4]. There are three common modes of presentation for SMD. It can be the initial presentation of a malignancy where the primary tumor has not yet been detected. In some cases, both primary and spine metastasis is detected at the same time, and in others, spinal metastasis detected after the treatment of the primary tumor may be years later. In certain cases, the primary tumor may be undetectable. The majority of spine metastases are detected in autopsy [5]. The order of incidence of primary tumors metastasizing to bone is prostate, breast, kidney, lung, and thyroid cancer. From autopsy studies, the incidence of skeletal metastasis for various primary tumors is as follows: breast, 68% (range of 33–85%); prostate cancer, 42% (range of 28–60%); thyroid cancer, 36% (range of 30–55%); lung cancer, 35% (range of 33–40%); kidney cancer, 6% (range of 5–7%); esophageal cancer, 5% (range of 3–11%); gastrointestinal tract cancers, 11% (range of 8–13%); and rectal cancer. Most cases of spinal metastasis are asymptomatic; hence, the exact prevalence is unknown [6].

Pathogenesis and Pathology

The primary neoplasm can reach the spine via the hematogenous spread, direct extension, or invasion from the adjacent lesion and rarely by seeding from the cerebrospinal fluid. The exact mechanism of intradural extramedullary metastasis is unknown. There are five mechanisms by which tumor cells can metastasize to the intradural extramedullary space alone or in combination. The spread from Batson's venous plexus, perineural lymphatics, seeding from local invasion adjacent to the dura, spread from subarachnoid space-drop metastasis or leptomeningeal spread, and hematogenous via the arterial system. The most common tumors spread through this method include lung, renal, thyroid, and primary bone tumors [7].

The most common mode of spread is hematogenous. The neoplastic cells from the primary site migrate or, through a process of neovascularization, attach to the basement membrane of the vessel wall. There, neoplastic cells disrupt the basement membrane by producing proteolytic enzymes (integrin/cadherin). Then, it spreads to distant sites hematogenous by attaching to the basement membrane of the vessels using proteolytic enzymes. In the distant target tissue, it destroys the basement membrane and becomes attached to it. The chemotactic factors and RANK ligand produced by tumor cells stimulate osteoclasts, leading to bone resorption. This continued growth and survival of the tumor cells destroys the cortical and cancellous bone in the metastatic site [8, 9]. Once within the vertebrae, the tumor cells produce cytokines that promote osteoclast-mediated osteolysis. This causes more release of tumor-promoting growth factors. This results in a cycle of destruction of both cortical and trabecular bone. The pain in SMD is due to endosteal nociceptor stimulation by periosteal stretching, inflammation, and tumor-related cytokines [10].

Presentations of a Patient with Spinal Metastatic Disease

Back pain is the most typical presentation of SMD. Pain during the night and rest are characteristic features. The pain can be local, radicular, or mechanical. Local pain is mostly due to periosteal stretching, increased endosteal pressure, and local inflammation due to tumor deposition. This pain is often felt at rest and exacerbated during the night. Often respond well to anti-inflammatory medications, steroids, and radiotherapy. Radicular pain is due to the compression of neural elements by the tumor tissue. This type of pain often follows a dermatomal distribution. This pain responds to steroids, chemotherapy, and radiotherapy [11]. The mechanical pain is due to instability. It is exacerbated by activity and is relieved with rest. There was no exacerbation during the night. Mechanical pain does not respond to analgesics, steroids, chemotherapy, or radiotherapy. The sudden onset of severe pain, which is exacerbated with movements and during the night, may indicate a pathological fracture [12].

SMD can cause epidural compression and neurological deficits. We have to perform a neurological evaluation of the patient. Motor, sensory, and autonomic functions need to be checked. Some patients may present with paraplegia or quadriplegia, while others may present with features of cauda equina syndrome. Compression fractures may lead to deformities of the spine [13].

There are various skeletal-related events (SREs) in SMD. SREs include pathological vertebral compression fractures, spinal cord or nerve root compression, hypercalcemia, and anemia. Increased bone turnover and bone resorption in metastatic disease lead to hypercalcemia. It is seen in approximately 30% of patients and indicates rapid progression of the disease. Hypercalcemia leads to weakness, vomiting, rhythm abnormalities of the heart, anorexia, renal disease, and coma. Hypercalcemia has a poor prognosis. Anemia is due to bone marrow suppression due to the tumor itself or to the effect of chemotherapy. SMD patients are at risk of coagulopathies. Neutropenia and thrombocytopenia are also seen. There is also an increased risk of DVT among SMD patients [14]. Women with breast and lung cancers and males with prostate and lung cancers are at high risk of developing SREs [15].

Mechanical Instability in SMD

Neoplastic spinal instability is defined as the loss of spinal integrity due to the neoplastic process. It results in movement-related pain, progressive deformity, or neurological deficits under physiological loading. Mechanical instability in SMD requires surgical stabilization or vertebral augmentation irrespective of the degree of epidural compression. Chemotherapy and radiation are ineffective in correcting instability [16]. The Spinal Oncology Study Group (SOSG) proposed criteria for assessing neoplastic spinal instability. It is known as the Spinal Instability Neoplastic Score (SINS) (Table 1). The estimation of instability in SINS is based on five objective radiographic criteria:

1. Location of the affected vertebrae in the spine
2. Type of lesion (lytic, sclerotic, or mixed)

3. Radiographic alignment of the spine
4. Vertebral body collapse
5. Involvement of posterolateral elements and a subjective symptom - Pain (Table 1).

Table 1. SINS scoring for metastatic spinal instability

Element of SINS	Score
Location	
Junctional (occiput-C2, C7–T2, T1 1–LI, L5–S1)	3
Mobile spine (C3–C6, L2–L4)	2
Semi-rigid (T3–T10)	1
Rigid (S2–S5)	0
Pain relief with recumbency and/or pain with movement/loading of the spine	
Yes	3
No (occasional pain but not mechanical)	1
Pain free lesion	0
Bone lesion	
Lytic	2
Mixed (lytic/blastic)	1
Blastic	0
Radiographic spinal alignment	
Subluxation/translation present	4
De novo deformity (kyphosis/scoliosis)	2
Normal alignment	0
Vertebral body collapse	
>50% collapse	3
<50% collapse	2
No collapse with >50% body involved	1
None of the above	0
Posterolateral involvement of the spinal elements (facet, pedicle or CV joint fracture or replacement with tumor)	
Bilateral	3
Unilateral	1
None of the above	0

Vertebral metastatic lesions with a low SINS score (0-6) are stable, and no surgical intervention is needed. A high SINS score (13-18) indicates unstable lesions and requires stabilization. Those with moderate scores (7-12) are potentially unstable. SINS has high inter- and intraobserver reliability [17]. SINS does not give any algorithm for treatment but helps the surgeon to identify those lesions at risk of progressive collapse. The disadvantage of SINS is that it does not consider the size and location of the lesion in the vertebra. Additionally, there is a large group that is potentially unstable (7-12). The size of the lytic SMD is related to its stability [18].

Attempts were made to incorporate the Dennis three-column concept used in traumatic fractures for assessing stability in SMD. However, they could not succeed, as the pattern of bony and soft tissue disruption in metastasis is entirely different from traumatic fractures. Intervertebral discs and ligaments are not involved in pathological fractures due to metastasis. The bony architecture is also different. The pathological fracture in the spine in metastatic diseases can be either a wedge compression fracture or a burst fracture. Wedge compression fractures are common in the dorsal spine and are due to flexion injury. Burst fractures are common in the cervical and lumbar spine in axial loading. The risk factors for vertebral instability in metastatic diseases include many factors. Increased axial rigidity, location of metastatic disease in the anterior third of the vertebral body in the sagittal plane and middle third in the axial plane, size of involvement in more than 55% of the vertebrae, and decreased bone density are all associated with increased instability. Costovertebral joint involvement, upper thoracic spine involvement in the dorsal region, and posterior element destruction in the dorsolumbar and lumbar spine increase instability [19].

SMD is a systemic disease that can lead to reduced bone density. Vertebral disease itself makes the vertebra prone to fractures. Both of these factors can lead to deformity and misalignment of the spine and cord compression. Malalignment of spinopelvic parameters such as pelvic retroversion and high pelvic tilt is associated with an increased risk of compression fractures [20].

There are no guidelines for the treatment of patients with indeterminate spinal instability (SINS 7 to 12). A study by Brian L et al. showed improved outcomes with the treatment of these patients and suggested discussing the risk and benefits to them before treatment. Surgical stabilization was associated with prolonged survival and ambulation in these patients compared to radiation alone. Cement augmentation with radiation has the lowest revision treatment with prolonged ambulation until death in the majority of their patients. Patients with radioresistant tumors with indeterminant stability should not be treated with external beam radiotherapy alone [21].

Neurological Involvement

Neurological involvement can result in sensory, motor, and autonomic dysfunction [22]. The Spine Oncology Study Group (SOSG) has described a grading system for assessing epidural compression: metastatic epidural spinal cord compression (MESCC). This grading utilizes the axial T2W image of the metastatic vertebra at the site of maximum compression. There are six grades of compression. A pure bone lesion is grade 0. A lesion impinging the epidural space is grade 1. It is divided into 1a- epidural impingement without deformation of the thecal sac. 1b- Deformation of the thecal sac without spinal cord abutment. 1c- Deformation of the thecal sac with spinal cord abutment but without cord compression. Grade 2 spinal cord compression but CSF visible around the cord. Grade 3 spinal cord compression with no CSF visible around the cord (Figure 1) [23].

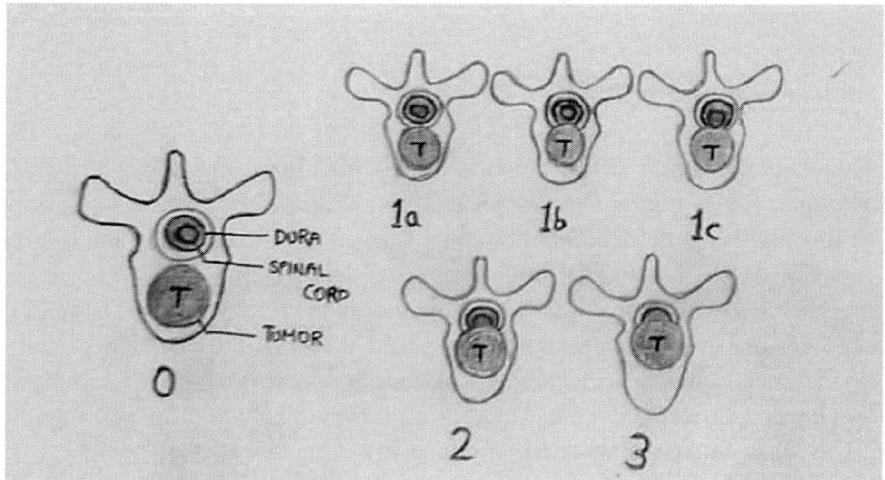

Figure 1. Diagrammatic representation of MESCC grades.

Metastatic spinal cord compression is an emergency. Untimely treatment can lead to paralysis. All tumors that metastasize to the spine may not cause epidural spinal cord compression. Prostate, breast, and lung cancers are common causes of MESCC (15-20%). Non-Hodgkin lymphoma, renal cell cancer, and multiple myeloma account for 5 to 10% of cases. The remainder is from colorectal cancers, sarcoma, and unknown primaries. MESCC may be the primary presentation in cases of rapidly growing cancers such as lung or breast cancer, but in others, it may be present after the detection of the primary tumor [24].

Paralysis in SMD is mainly due to instability and spinal cord compression. Approximately 5 to 15% of cancer patients can develop spinal cord compression. Paralysis develops according to the grade of spinal cord compression. MRI is the most sensitive imaging modality for identifying spinal cord compression. Even the findings of cord compression in MRI may not correlate with the degree of paralysis. The degree of paralysis depends on the level of the lesion. Neurological deficits can be assessed using the American Spinal Cord Injury Association (ASIA) scale. The severity of paralysis does not correlate with the MESCC scale. More than half of patients with grade 1b or more compression at the C1-D2 level and grade 1c or more compression at D3 to D5 develop worse paralysis. Patients with anterolateral or circumferential MESCC grade 2 or 3 compressions at C7-D1 1 can develop rapidly progressive paralysis [25]. MESCC causes spinal cord damage by direct compression or by vascular occlusion [26].

Histology of Tumors

The oncologic status of the tumor depends mainly on histology. Histology determines the aggressiveness of the tumor and its response to various treatments. The other factors to be considered in the oncological status are the extent of the disease and previous treatments.

Histology is the most important predictor of survival in SMD. The tumors can be slow growing (breast, prostate, and thyroid). intermediate growing (kidney and uterus) and rapidly growing tumors (lung, liver, stomach, esophagus, pancreas, sarcomas, and tumors with unknown primary). Rapidly growing tumors have the worst prognosis [27].

According to histology, certain tumor types are amenable to systemic chemotherapy. It may take some time for the effect of chemotherapy to appear. Hence, chemotherapy is reserved for asymptomatic or minimally symptomatic patients. For hematological malignancies and Ewing's disease, sarcoma chemotherapy is highly effective, although they are aggressive tumors. Metastasis from breast and prostate cancers can be treated with chemotherapy. We have to avoid chemotherapy in patients with spinal instability and neurological deficits.

Certain tumors are radiosensitive. The problem with radiotherapy is the presence of the spinal cord in the field. The dose of radiation used should be within the safety limit for the spinal cord when conventional radiotherapy is used. Tumors that respond favorably to this dose of radiation are considered radiosensitive. Myeloma, lymphoma, and seminoma are highly radiosensitive. SMDs from breast, prostate, ovary, and neuroendocrine tumors are radiosensitive. Sarcomas, renal cell carcinoma, non-small cell tumors of the lung, thyroid malignancies, melanoma, and hepatocellular carcinomas are radioresistant tumors [28].

Highly vascular metastases, such as renal cell carcinoma, thyroid carcinoma, hepatocellular carcinoma, melanoma, and giant cell tumors, can bleed profusely during surgery. Preoperative embolization can be effective in controlling bleeding during surgery [29].

The extent of visceral involvement also determines survival. Patients with extensive visceral disease have poor survival. Surgery in such patients may have poor outcomes. Lung metastasis causes decreased pulmonary function, and liver metastasis can lead to bleeding tendencies, making such patients poor candidates for surgical treatment. Staging of the disease is mandatory in all patients before surgery.

Prognostic Staging of SMD

There are many classification-based prognostic staging systems for SMD (Table 2). They all estimate the survival of patients with SMD.

Table 2. Factors considered in different prognostic scoring systems for SMD (Modified from Ref. [30])

Classification	Primary tumor	Performance status	No. of vertebral Mets	Bone Mets	Visceral Mets	Previous treatments	others
Modified Bauer	Y			Y	Y		
Tomita	Y			Y	Y		
Revised Tokuhashi	Y	Y	Y	Y	Y		
Revised Katagiri	Y	Y		Y	Y	Y	Brain metastasis, WBC, Hb, platelet, albumin, bilirubin, CRP, LDH
NESMS	Y	Y		Y	Y	Y	Serum albumin
SORG	Y	Y	Y		Y	Y	Age, WBC, Hb, brain metastasis

(WBC, white blood cell; Hb, hemoglobin; CRP, C-reactive protein; LDH, lactate dehydrogenase; NESMS, New England Spinal Metastasis Score; SORG, Spine Oncology Research Group)

Life expectancy is assessed using the total prognostic scores calculated by adding the scores of individual prognostic factors. Different factors are considered in each scoring system. The scoring helps the surgeon to assess the life expectancy of the patient and decide on surgical management. However, recent studies have shown poor accuracy for such prognostic scoring systems [30].

Even though the nature and extent of previous treatment may influence the oncologic status, it may be difficult to stratify or quantify it. We have to consider it on an individual basis. The responses to previous treatments will affect the further treatment of SMD. A multidisciplinary approach with persons from medical oncology, radiation oncology, and surgical teams is necessary for developing a treatment plan.

NOMS

It is a decision-making framework for SMD developed by a multidisciplinary spine team at Memorial Sloan-Kettering Cancer Center (MSKCC) (Appendix 1). The four fundamental assessments in the NOMS are neurologic, oncologic, mechanical instability, and systemic disease, which we have discussed above. It helps the surgeon make a decision regarding the management of SMD based on these four cardinal points. They can determine if the patients need surgery, radiotherapy, and/or chemotherapy [31].

Neurologic (MESSC)	Oncologic (Radiosensitive or resistant)	Mechanical Instability (SINS)	Systemic factor (Risk for surgery)	Treatment Options
Low grade	Yes	Stable		cEBRT
		Not stable		Surgery(stabilization) + cEBRT
	No	stable		SBRT
		Not stable		Surgery(stabilization) + SBRT
High grade	Yes	Stable		cEBRT
	No	Not stable		Surgery(stabilization) + cEBRT
		Stable		Separation surgery + SBRT
		Not stable		Surgery(stabilization) + cEBRT

Appendix 1. Treatment algorithm based on NOMS.

The neurologic consideration is the degree of epidural compression, myelopathy, or functional radiculopathy. The expected response and durability to conventional external beam radiation, stereotactic radiation surgery, chemotherapy, immunotherapy, or hormonal therapy are considerations in the oncologic part. Mechanical stability deals with pathologic fractures and their management, such as braces, cement augmentations, and percutaneous or open surgery for stabilization. The last consideration is given to systemic disease and medical comorbidities. The ability of the patient to tolerate the proposed treatment. For expected survival, if the expected expectancy is less than three months, surgical interventions should be avoided [32].

In the absence of mechanical instability, patients with highly radiosensitive tumors such as lymphoma, myeloma, and seminoma can be treated with radiation alone even in high-grade spinal cord compression (MESCC grade 2 or 3). This is due to their rapid response to radiotherapy or chemotherapy. Patients without mechanical instability grade 0,1a, 1b can be treated with radiation alone as an initial method. High-grade tumors (MESCC 2 and 3) that are not radiosensitive are treated by surgical decompression followed by radiotherapy. For grade 1c, the role of radiotherapy or surgery is not clearly defined. High-dose hypofractionated radiation or SRS may be administered to avoid spinal cord toxicity [33].

The oncological assessment is based on the histology of tumors and their responsiveness to presently available treatment methods. Radiotherapy is the most common mode of treatment used for SMD. Metastatic tumors are divided into radiosensitive and radioresistant tumors based on their response to conventional external beam radiotherapy (cEBRT). However, the problem with cEBRT is the radiation hazard to the spinal cord. Recent techniques such as image-guided radiation therapy (IGRT) help to give a precise dose of radiation to the tumor site without harming the spinal cord. Stereotactic radiosurgery (SRS) uses the IGRT platform and helps to administer a high dose of radiation in focused areas in a single fraction or 3 to 5 fractions.

Irrespective of MESSC grading, radiosensitive tumors can be treated with cEBRT. It can provide local tumor control and pain relief. CEBRT improves the ambulatory status of the patient. Low-grade radioresistant tumors with MESCC grades 0, 1a, and 1b can be treated with IGRT alone without the need for surgical decompression. Radioresistant tumors with high-grade epidural cord compression require surgical decompression and stabilization before IGRT can be administered. The goals of surgery are the restoration of mechanical stability, circumferential decompression of the spinal cord, and prevention of spinal cord damage and neurological deficits during radiation. The maximum safe dose of radiation to the spinal cord without damage is 14 Gy. The minimum effective dose for tumor destruction in SRS is 15 Gy. To safely give more than 15G circumferential separation of 2-3 mm of issues between the tumor and spinal cord is needed [30, 34, 35].

Irrespective of the MESCC compression and radiosensitivity, mechanical instability is an independent factor for surgical stabilization or cement augmentation. Patients with mechanical instability are presented with movement-related pain. The SINS helps to assess spinal instability in SMD. A SINS between 13 and 18 is an indication of surgical stabilization. Painful compression fractures in the absence of mechanical spinal instability or significant posterior element involvement can be treated with a cement augmentation procedure.

The systemic factors depend on tumor histology, the extent of spinal and visceral metastasis, and associated medical comorbidities. All these factors predict the survival of the patient. The prediction of treatment methods is based on life expectancy and the ability of the patient to tolerate the specific treatment modality. Surgical interventions must be avoided in patients with aggressive tumors because of shorter survival. Preoperative staging helps to determine the systemic factors and whether surgery is feasible in a particular case.

LMNOP

It is a newer algorithm for decision-making in SMD. It incorporates factors such as location and levels of spinal disease (L), mechanical instability (M), neurology (N), oncology (O), patient fitness, prognosis, patient wishes, and previous treatments (P). The LMNOP addresses 3 factors that were not given due consideration in the NOMS. The location of the lesion, whether in the anterior or posterior column, the number of levels involved, and whether they are contiguous or noncontiguous, were considered in this system. The LMNOP is a decision-making system integrated with SINS.

In the craniocervical region, instability can present with severe mechanical pain before producing neurological deficits. This is due to the large spinal canal in this area. Occepetocervical fusion can be performed for such cases. For the subaxial spine between C3 and C6, anterior corpectomy with cage and plate fixation for a single level and combined anterior and posterior fixation can be performed in multilevel disease. An anterior approach is not feasible for the upper thoracic spine (D2-D5). A lateral extracavitory approach or costotranversectomy is more feasible. Costotranversectomy and the extracavitory lateral approach are preferred in the lower thoracic spine through anterior, posterior, or combined approaches. The reconstruction of vertebral bodies is performed using autografts, allografts, metallic cages, or polymethyl methacrylate cement. Stabilization can be performed using anterior or posterior instrumentation. The lumbar and lumbosacral regions can be fixed using all posterior or combined anterior or posterior approaches.

Other than in the suboccipital region, SMD usually produces kyphotic deformities. In the suboccipital region, it can produce translational and rotational deformities. In the dorsal spine chest wall disruption, destruction of the pedicle, costovertebral joints, facets, and pedicle can cause kyphoscoliotic deformities. The deformities due to metastatic disease are flexible and can be corrected by positioning themselves. Verebrectomy and reconstruction can correct the deformities. Shortening of the spine by compression after removal of the tumor is another technique for correction of the deformities. Fusion procedures are not required in SMD. There is less chance of bony fusion in SMD. There are many reasons for this, such as reduced life expectancy, the use of adjunct chemotherapy and radiotherapy compromising the local environment for fusion and associated medical comorbidities and poor nutrition [36].

Imaging in Spine Metastasis

Imaging studies in the spine's metastatic disease aim to find the lesion at the earliest. They help to differentiate it from other pathologies. It is also helpful to determine the size and extent of the lesion, including skip lesions in the spine and other visceral metastases. Epidural and extraspinal extensions can be assessed by imaging. We can take biopsies and plan treatment by assessing the images.

Plain radiographs are the initial investigation. A plain X-ray detects a lesion when it is more than 2 cm in size or when more than 50% of the cancellous bone is destroyed. Up to 40% of cases are missed in routine radiographic evaluation. Epidural lesions may show erosion of the posterior border of the vertebra. The destruction of the pedicle - the ``winking owl sign`` can be seen [37]. Computerized tomography scans can detect smaller lesions and both osteolytic and sclerotic lesions. It can detect metastatic spinal disease

6 months earlier than a plain X-ray. It can detect cortical destruction. The epidural mass may present as amorphous soft tissue displacing the thecal sac or filling the neural foramen. CT myelography is useful when an MRI scan is contraindicated [38].

The FGD PET/CT scan has sensitivity similar to an MRI scan. PET scans are more sensitive than bone scans for detecting metastasis from lung and lymphoma. FGD PET scans are more sensitive for detecting osteolytic lesions than osteosclerotic lesions. It can also differentiate between osteoporotic compression fractures and malignant pathological fractures in FGD avid tumors. However, its sensitivity is low for smaller lesions and those with lower metabolic activity. Bone scintigraphy shows hot spots in the majority of metastatic lesions. However, it will show cold areas in myeloma, leukemia, anaplastic carcinoma, and highly malignant tumors due to reduced blood flow or the absence of reactive new bone formation. A bone scan is nonspecific for the detection of spine metastasis, as fractures and degenerative changes and healed lesions after radiotherapy may show increased uptake [30].

MRI scan is the most sensitive (98%) investigation. It can detect early lesions before trabecular or cortical bone destruction. The red marrow to yellow marrow conversion in adults occurs from the center to the periphery of the vertebral body. In normal T1WI, the red marrow is hyperintense but hypointense relative to the intervertebral disc and muscle in metastatic diseases. The STIR sequence is the most sensitive sequence for spinal metastasis because of the high contrast between hyperintense tumors and suppressed marrow tissue. The presence of an epidural soft tissue mass and the convex posterior vertebral border is 99% specific for metastatic vertebral compression fractures. In T2WI, there will be hyperintensity of tumor tissue compared to the marrow and a break in the black line representing the posterior vertebral border [40]. A CT scan and MRI imaging can differentiate pre-lytic, lytic, and sclerotic secondaries. Extraosseous soft tissue, intradural extension, and neural compression can also be identified by these imaging modalities. The sternum plays an essential role in the stability of the dorsal spine by providing attachment to the ribs. Pathological fractures of the sternum in SMD can lead to instability and kyphosis. The sternum must be included in the radiological evaluation of SMD [5, 38].

The role of tumor markers in the diagnosis of SMD is limited. They are useful to rule out multiple myeloma and primary bone tumors. Beta 2 microglobulin is used as a marker for multiple myeloma. The commonly used biochemical markers for various tumors include CA 19.9 (pancreatic, gallbladder, and bile duct cancers), CA 15.3/CA27.29 (breast), CEA (colorectal and breast), CA 125 (ovarian cancer), PSA (prostate) and calcitonin (medullary carcinoma thyroid) [41].

Histopathological confirmation is mandatory in all cases of SMD to rule out similar lesions, such as infections. A biopsy helps to identify radiosensitive tumors. Fine needle aspiration cytology (FNAC) is sufficient when we know the site of the primary lesion. In cases of unknown primary, an image-guided (CT/X-ray) or an open biopsy can be performed [42].

Management of Spinal Metastasis

The goal of the management of SMD is palliation. Control of pain, preservation or restoration of neurological functions, maintaining spinal stability, and improving quality of life are the aims of treatment. There are nonoperative and operative options available.

Nonoperative Treatment

Treating pain is the most important part of nonoperative management. Analgesics, steroids, bisphosphonates, denosumab, and hormonal therapy are the common drugs used. Opioids, NSAIDs, and steroids help to reduce tumor-related local pain and radicular pain. Buccal, sublingual, or intranasal fentanyl can be used for effective pain relief. Intrathecal infiltration of analgesics is effective when higher doses of opioids are required for analgesia. Therapeutic nerve blocks are also effective. Steroids can reduce edema and compression of neural structures and reduce pain [43]. For chronic pain, due to SMD, various modalities are being tried. Chronic pain in the majority is due to the neuropathic type. Spinal cord stimulation can be performed to relieve pain. Nerve block procedures such as paravertebral nerve block, erector spinal blocks, medial branch blocks, and epidural steroid injections are being used, but literature support is lacking [44].

Bisphosphonates such as zoledronic acid help to control skeletally related events such as hypercalcemia and vertebral compression fractures. Denosumab, a fully human monoclonal antibody, is superior to zoledronic acid in preventing or delaying SREs. It is also useful in reducing treatment-related secondary osteoporosis in the breast and prostate [45].

Chemotherapy helps in the systemic and local control of the primary tumor. Chemotherapy is effective in multiple myeloma and hematological malignancies. They help to reduce morbidity. Secondaries from breast and prostate carcinoma can be treated using hormonal therapy [46].

Percutaneous Interventions

Percutaneous interventions such as vertebral augmentation and vertebral tumor ablative therapy are also used for pain relief, increasing stability, and local tumor control.

Vertebroplasty and Kyphoplasty

Minimally invasive procedures can be used to treat SMD. These techniques result in less trauma to soft tissues, minimal blood loss, and shorter hospital stays. The overall mortality is very low compared to surgery. Vertebroplasty and kyphoplasty are two minimally invasive procedures used in SMD. Vertebroplasty injects bone cement into the vertebral body under image guidance. Kyphoplasty is a balloon-assisted vertebroplasty. Here, an inflatable bone tamp is created to restore the shape of the vertebra. It allows controlled low-pressure cement injection into previously created cavities. It also reduces cement leakage and other complications associated with vertebroplasty. These procedures are indicated for those who are not ideal candidates for spine surgery due to a lifespan of fewer than three months. Local infection is an absolute contraindication. Coagulopathies and allergies are other contra-indications [47].

Vertebral tumor ablative therapy is used in conjunction with vertebral augmentation procedures. They are helpful in additional pain relief and local tumor control. Radiofrequency, microwave, and cryoablation are commonly used. Radiofrequency (RF) and microwaves cause coagulation necrosis of the tumor by creating heat in the local tumor environment. Cryoablation uses argon gas, which rapidly cools and results in a decrease in temperature to approximately $-100°C$, resulting in tissue death. This technique is typically employed when there is an extraosseous extension of the tumor into surrounding soft tissues. Vertebral augmentation follows ablative therapy. This combined therapy has shown increased pain relief. This method can be used in patients who are poor candidates for open surgery and those with a life expectancy of less than three months [48].

Radiotherapy

Radiotherapy is an effective method for the palliation of painful bone metastasis. It gives complete relief of pain with minimal complications in one-third of patients. Conventional external beam radiation (cEBRT) uses both short-course and long-course radiation regimens. In a short course regimen, 30 G radiation is given in 10 divided fractions. In the long course, regiment 20G is divided into 5 fractions or 8 G in a single fraction. Studies have demonstrated equal results for both short- and long-course regimens. Single-dose radiation has higher retreatment rates.

The choice of regimen depends on the survival of the patient. If the expected survival is poor, then short-course radiation is recommended, and a long course is advised for patients with good long-term survival [19]. Although multi-fraction radiation was given for those patients with spinal cord compression, no data are supporting its superiority. Doses beyond 30 G in 10 fractions do not affect motor functions or the local control of spinal cord compression in radioresistant tumors. 30 G in 10 divided fractions is considered the standard treatment for spinal metastasis with epidural compression. Retreatment radiation can be given for painful spine metastasis. It has been shown to improve motor functions. The improvement of motor functions after reradiation depends on the effectiveness of initial radiation, performance status, period of development of motor deficits, and visceral metastasis. The radiotherapy schedule does not affect motor recovery [49].

There is also a role for radiation after surgery. The ambulatory ability of patients who received radiotherapy was significantly greater than that of patients who received radiotherapy following surgery. The walking ability of patients who underwent surgery alone was greater than that of patients who underwent radiotherapy alone. There is controversy regarding the timing of radiation following surgery [50]. The main factors determining wound healing following surgery after radiation are the interval between radiation and surgery and the total dose of radiation. Radiotherapy decreases the tensile strength of the wound after surgery. If radiotherapy is given immediately after surgery, the inflammatory response is inhibited, and the number of inflammatory cells in the wound site is reduced, affecting wound healing. There must be at least a week interval following radiotherapy for surgery. Radiotherapy can be given safely after a week following surgery [51].

Permanent radiation injury to the spinal cord is a dreaded complication of radiation therapy for SMD. There is no effective treatment for this condition. There are three forms of radiation myelopathy. An acute and rapid onset lower motor neuron paralysis. The second type is a transient variety characterized by a positive Lhermitte's sign, and the third variety is delayed progressive paralysis. The thoracic cord has the least tolerance to radiation [52].

Stereotactic BT

cEBRT was the mainstay of treatment for spinal metastasis for a long time. However, the limited dose of radiation that can be given through this route without risking the adjacent organs is a disadvantage of cEBRT. Stereotactic body radiotherapy (SBRT) is a highly conformal radiation therapy that delivers a high dose of radiation with precision to the target area without affecting the spinal cord. It can be administered safely and effectively. It is also effective for local control of radioresistant spinal metastasis. Single-fraction SBRT is more effective for local control than higher fractions. However, a single fraction has a higher incidence of vertebral compression fractures than multiple doses. SBRT can provide greater pain relief than cEBRT [53].

There are many guidelines for selecting patients with spinal metastasis for SBRT. In general, patients with a solid metastatic lesion in the spine or paraspinal region with 3 or fewer contiguous segments, low-grade epidural compression, a relatively stable spine, limited systemic disease, and a life expectancy of at least 3 months are ideal for SBRT. The absolute contraindications are spinal instability and high-grade epidural compression. In patients with highly radiosensitive and chemosensitive tumors such as multiple myeloma, lymphoma, and seminoma, cEBRT is the preferred method of radiation. SBRT can be used as an effective adjuvant postoperative therapy following minimally invasive and open surgeries. It has a few complications, including vertebral compression fractures [54].

SBRT and cEBRT are some complications. The metastatic spine is prone to vertebral compression fractures. Lytic vertebral lesions are more prone to compression fractures. However, sclerotic lesions are also prone to skeletally-related events. SBRT will make the metastatic spine more prone to compression fractures than cEBRT. There is a transient increase in bone pain during or shortly after conventional radiotherapy called pain flare. Pain flares can be seen in SBRT. We can suspect pain flares when there is a 2-point increase in the worst pain score on the BPI (Brief Pain Inventory) with no change in oral morphine equivalent dose OR a 25% increase in oral morphine equivalent dose with no decrease in worst pain score OR any initiation of steroid therapy. The esophagus is closely related to the thoracic vertebrae; hence, there is a high risk of radiation-induced esophagitis during radiotherapy. Although rare in SBRT radiation, myelopathy, plexopathy, and radiculopathy can occur with cEBRT [55].

Surgical Treatment

The goal of the treatment of spinal metastasis is palliation. There are very rare cases of SMD, such as isolated cases of renal cell carcinoma metastasis, where we can obtain a complete cure. The main indications for surgery in SMD are uncontrollable pain, neurological deficits, mechanical instability, and radioresistant tumors with high-grade epidural compression. Surgery is considered when the estimated life expectancy is more than three months. The aims of surgery in SMD are to correct the deformity or to prevent it. With instrumentation, we can stabilize the mechanically unstable spine. In cases of neurological deficits, surgery helps to decompress the spinal cord and nerve roots.

Laminectomy has been used to treat SMD for a long time and helps to decompress neurological structures. Later laminectomy followed by radiotherapy was found to be more effective than surgery alone. However, laminectomy alone is not a preferred option for SMD due to complications such as acceleration of existing spinal instability and wound complications [56].

With advancements in spine surgery, we can now reach the vertebral body from either posterior or anterior or combined approaches. The vertebral body is the site of the lesion in most cases. Direct posterior, posterolateral, and anterior approaches help the surgeon decompress the spine at 360 degrees. Neurological recovery depends on the preoperative neurological status, rapidity of neurological deterioration, and duration.

Surgery can give better results than radiotherapy alone. Surgery followed by radiation gives better results. Surgical treatment is also associated with complications such as wound problems, CSF fistula, deterioration of existing neurological deficits, the appearance of new deficits, implant-related complications, and medical problems such as pneumonia and bleeding [57].

Surgery for SMD aims at oncological cure, spinal stabilization, neurological palliation, pain relief, and biopsy for diagnosis. The Ennecking system was first introduced to the concept of surgical margins in the treatment of primary tumors. The various levels include intralesional, which is a debulking procedure without taking the margins. Marginal where the excision of the tumor along the pseudo capsule in the reactive zone, the satellite and skip lesions are not included. Wide excision also includes the satellite lesions in the excision. This includes a few centimeters of normal tissues also.

Radicle resection involves the excision of the entire compartment, including skip lesions. Unless in radicle resection, we cannot ensure complete clearance of the tumor. Hence, in other forms of resection in high-grade malignancies, Ennecking recommends adjuvant treatment using radiation or chemotherapy to reduce recurrence. Radicle margins are not feasible in the vertebrae, although marginal and wide resections can be performed. In SMD, individual vertebrae can be considered a compartment. The barriers preventing the spread of the tumor are the periosteum covering the vertebrae, the intervertebral disc, and ligaments (ALL, PLL, ligamentum flavum, supra, and interspinous ligaments). The usual site of tumor invasion occurs through the lateral periosteum and PLL. In the PLL, the lateral area is thin compared to the central region, and the most likely route of vertical extension is the lateral periosteum [58].

Radiological staging is important for the analysis of the extent of the lesion and the plan of the surgery. The Tomita classification is one of the earliest classifications that divides the lesions into intracompartmental, extracompartmental, and multiple (Figure 2).

Weinstein Boriani and Biagini's classification is an extensively used staging system. In this, the vertebra is divided into 12 equal zones in the transverse plane. There are five layers in the transverse plain: extraosseous soft tissues, intraosseous superficial, intraosseous deep, extraosseous (extradural), and extraosseous (intradural). The vertebral artery is considered a separate layer. The longitudinal extent is based on the vertebral segments involved. This system helps the surgeon perform surgery according to oncological margins (Figure 3) [59, 60].

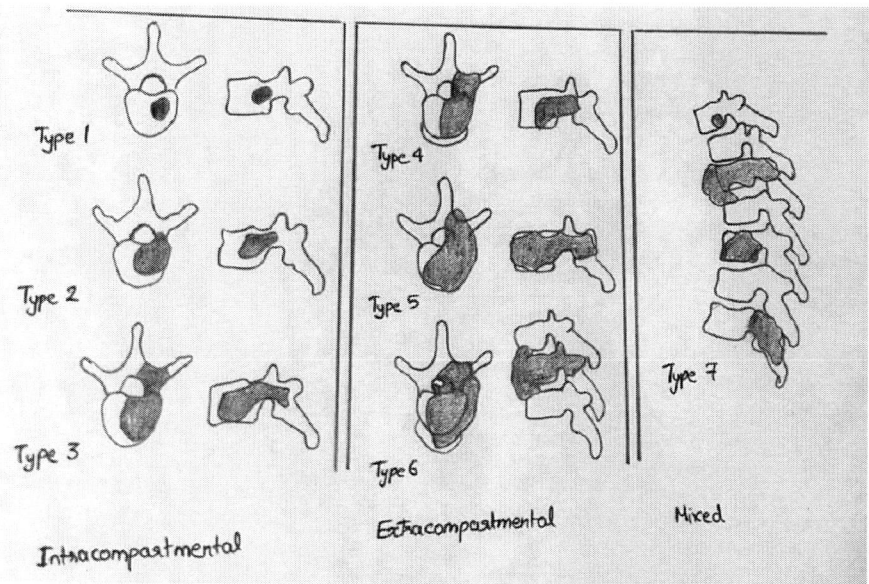

Figure 2. Tomita classification. *Intracompartmental*: Type 1 lesion confined to the vertebral body; Type 2 lesion extending to the pedicle; Type 3 lesion extending to posterior elements. *Extracompartmental*: Type 4 spinal canal extension; Type 5 paravertebral extension; Type 6 lesion extending to the adjacent vertebra. *Multiple lesion*: Type 7 lesion involving multiple vertebrae.

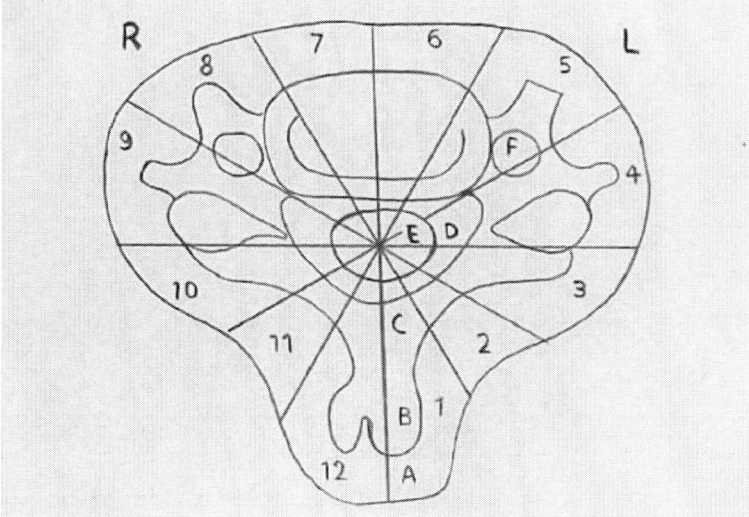

Figure 3. Weinstein Boriani and Biagini's classification.

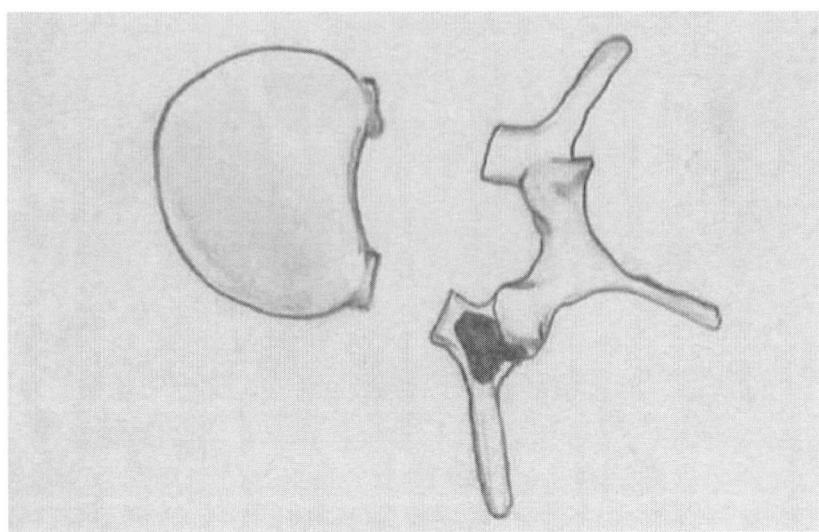

Figure 4. Diagrammatic representation of posterior arch resection where all the posterior elements of the vertebra are removed in toto.

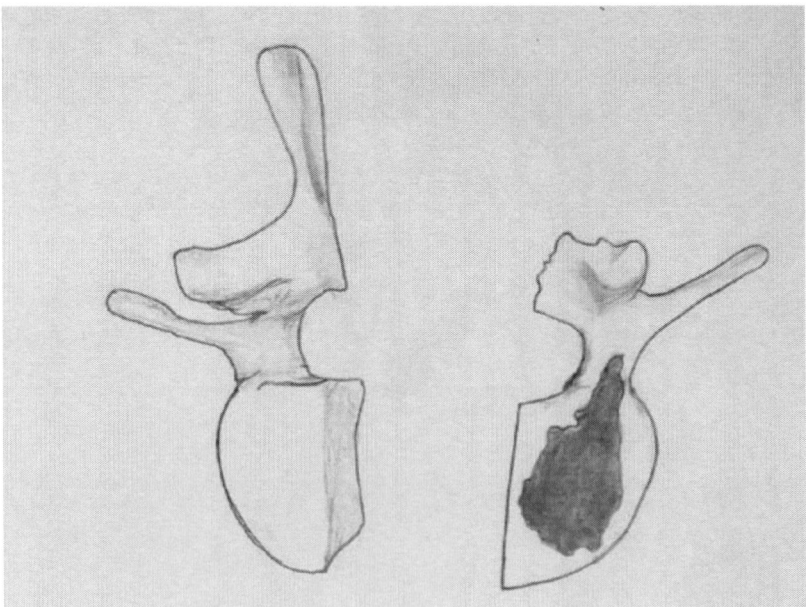

Figure 5. Image showing sagittal resection where the involved part of the body and posterior elements of the vertebra is removed. This is done in eccentrically located lesions in the vertebral body.

Depending on the location of the lesion, there are three main methods of en-bloc resection in the thoracolumbar spine: They are posterior arch resections where the posterior elements are removed in toto (Figure 4). This is done when the lesion is confined to the posterior element alone. Sagittal resection is performed for lesions confined eccentrically in the vertebral body (Figure 5). Vertebrectomy is performed for a lesion in the vertebral body. Enbloc spondylectomy decreases local recurrence and increases long-term survival in patients with SMD (Figure 6). It is the treatment of choice in patients with solitary or oligometastatic SMD [29].

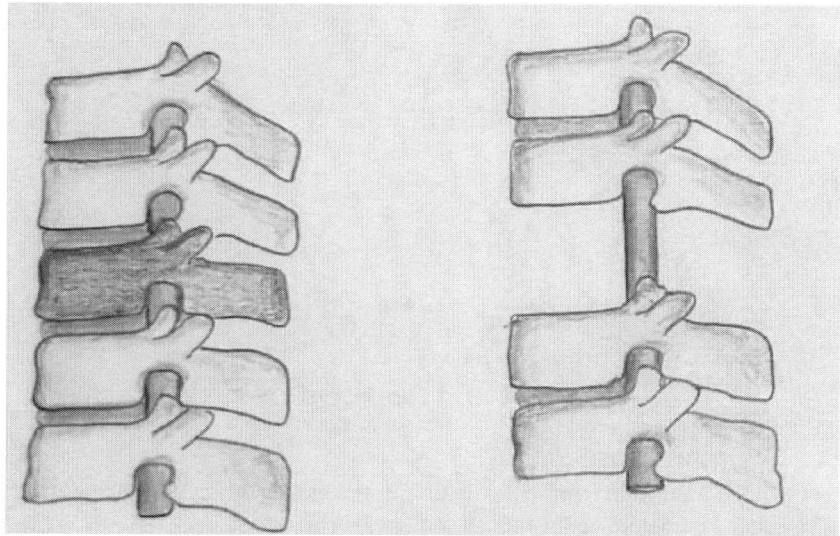

Figure 6. Diagrammatic representation of vertebrectomy where the entire vertebral body and posterior elements are removed and reconstruction of the body is performed using cages and bone grafts.

Separation Surgery

Separation surgery involves circumferential decompression of the spinal cord and nerve roots (Figure 7). It helps to preserve or restore neurological functions. It also helps to create a safe zone around the spinal cord for stereotactic radiotherapy (SBRT). The posterolateral or transpedicular approach is commonly used for separation surgery. It helps in the reexpansion of neural elements with 2 to 3 mm of space between the tumor and the spinal cord. Anterior decompression is the most difficult part of separation surgery [62].

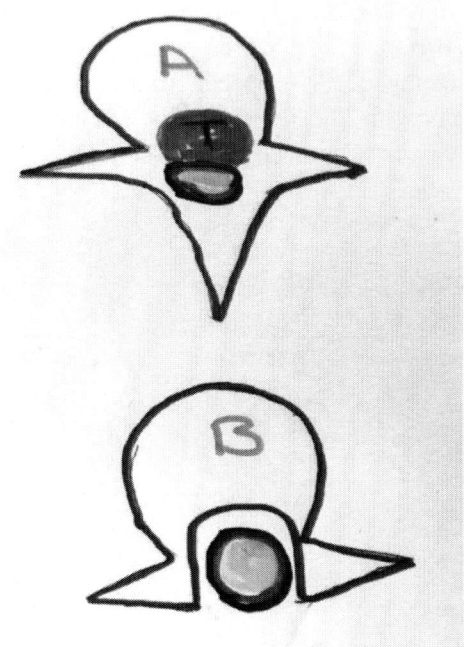

Figure 7. Diagrammatic representation of the vertebral lesion and its relation to the spinal cord before treatment (A) and after separation surgery (B).

Minimally Invasive Spine Surgery for Spinal Metastasis

Minimally invasive spine surgery techniques can be used in SMD. MISS can be used for biopsy, stabilization of an unstable spine, decompression, and separation surgery. It can give similar improvements in pain relief and neurological functions compared to conventional surgery. It has low morbidity, less blood loss, and a shorter operative time. However, the evidence for its use in SMD is low [62].

Conclusion

The incidence of spinal metastatic disease is increasing. Palliative therapy is our aim. Recent advancements in radiotherapy and surgical techniques have improved the outcomes of spinal metastasis. The strategies are still evolving, and better techniques are expected in the future.

References

[1] White, Andrew P., Md, Kwon, Brian K., Md, Phd, Frcsc, Lindskog, Dieter M., Md, Friedlaender, Gary E., Md, and Grauer, Jonathan N. Md. (October 2006). metastatic disease of the spine. *Journal of the American Academy of Orthopedic Surgeons*, 14, Issue 11, pp. 587-598.

[2] Van Den Brande, R., Mj Cornips, E., Peeters, M., Ost, P., Billiet, C., and Van De Kelft, E. (2022). epidemiology of spinal metastases, metastatic epidural spinal cord compression and pathologic vertebral compression fractures in patients with solid tumors: A systematic review. *Journal Of Bone Oncology.*, 35, 100446. Doi:10.10 16/J.Jbo.2022.100446.

[3] Steinberger, J. M., Yuk, F., Doshi, A. H., Green, S., and Germano, I. M. (2020). *Multidisciplinary Management of Metastatic Spine Disease: Initial Symptom-Directed Management.*, 7(Supplement_1), I33-I44. Doi:10.1093/Nop/Npaa048.

[4] Algra, P. R., Heimans, J. J., Valk, J., Nauta, J. J., Lachniet, M., and Van Kooten, B. (1992). Do metastases in vertebrae begin in the body or the pedicles? Imaging Study In 45 Patients. *American Journal of Roentgenology.*, 158(6), 1275-1279. Doi:10.221 4/Ajr.158.6.1590123.

[5] Zacharia, B., Subramaniam, D., and Joy, J. (2018 Mar). Skeletal metastasis-An epidemiological study. *Indian J Surg Oncol.*, 9(1), 46-51. Doi: 10.1007/S13193-01 7-0706-6. Epub 2017 Sep 28.

[6] Maccauro, G., Spinelli, M. S., Mauro, S., Perisano, C., Graci, C., and Rosa, M. A. (2011). Physiopathology of spine metastasis. *International Journal of Surgical Oncology.*, 2011, 1-8. Doi:10.1155/2011/107969.

[7] Land, C. F., Bowden, B. D., Morpeth, B. G., and Devine, J. G. (2019 May). Intradural extramedullary metastasis: A review of literature and case report. *Spinal Cord Ser Cases.*, 8, 5, 41. Doi: 10.1038/S41394-019-0181-0. Pmid: 31632701; Pmcid: Pmc6786287.

[8] Wiltse, L. L., Fonseca, A. S., Amster, J., Dimartino, P., and Ravessoud, F. A. (1993 Jun). relationship of the dura, hofmann's ligaments, batson's plexus, and a fibrovascular membrane lying on the posterior surface of the vertebral bodies and attaching to the deep layer of the posterior longitudinal ligament. an anatomical, radiologic, and clinical study. *Spine (Phila Pa 1976).*, 15, 18(8), 1030-43. Doi: 10.1097/00007632-199306150-00013.

[9] Mundy Gr. (2002). Metastasis to bone: causes, consequences and therapeutic opportunities. *Nat Rev Cancer*, 2, 584–593

[10] Wallace, A. N., Greenwood, T. J., and Jennings, J. W. (2015). Use of imaging in the management of metastatic spine disease with percutaneous ablation and vertebral augmentation. *American Journal of Roentgenology*, 205(2), 434–441. doi:10.2214/ajr.14.14199

[11] Helweg-Larsen, S., and Sørensen, P. S. (1994). Symptoms and signs in metastatic spinal cord compression: a study of progression from first symptom until diagnosis in 153 patients. *European Journal of Cancer.*, 30(3), 396-398. Doi:10.1016/0959-8049(94)90263-1.

[12] Planchard, R. F., Lubelski, D., Ehersman, J., et al. (2021). Surgical stabilization for patients with mechanical back pain secondary to metastatic spinal disease is associated with improved objective mobility metrics: Preliminary analysis in a cohort of 26 patients. *World Neurosurgery.*, 153, E28-E35. Doi:10.1016/J.Wneu.2021.06.034.

[13] Constans, J. P., De Divitiis, E., Donzelli, R., Spaziante, R., Meder, J. F., and Haye, C. (1983). Spinal metastases with neurological manifestations. *Journal Of Neurosurgery*, 59(1), 111–118. Doi:10.3171/Jns.1983.59.1.0111.

[14] Steinberger, J. M., Yuk, F., Doshi, A. H., Green, S., and Germano, I. M. (2020). *Multidisciplinary Management of Metastatic Spine Disease: Initial Symptom-Directed Management.*, 7(Supplement_1), I33-I44. Doi:10.1093/Nop/Npaa048.

[15] Herget, G., Saravi, B., Schwarzkopf, E., et al. (2021). Clinicopathologic characteristics, metastasis-free survival, and skeletal-related events in 628 patients with skeletal metastases in a tertiary orthopedic and trauma center. *World J Surg Onc.*, 19(1). Doi:10.1186/S12957-021-02169-7.

[16] Dakson, A., Leck, E., Brandman, D. M., and Christie, S. D. (2020). The clinical utility of the spinal instability neoplastic score (sins) system in spinal epidural metastases: A retrospective study. *Spinal Cord*, 58, 892–899.. Doi:10.1038/S41393-020-0432-8.

[17] Fisher, C. G., Versteeg, A. L., Schouten, R., Boriani, S., Varga, P. P., Rhines, L. D., Heran, M. K., Kawahara, N., Fourney, D., Reynolds, J. J., Fehlings, M. G, and Gokaslan, Z. L. (2014 Oct). Reliability of the spinal instability neoplastic scale among radiologists: an assessment of instability secondary to spinal metastases. *Ajr Am J Roentgenol.*, 203(4), 869-74. Doi: 10.2214/Ajr.13.12269.

[18] Palanca, M., Barbanti-Bròdano, G., Marras, D., et al. (2021). Type, size, and position of metastatic lesions explain the deformation of the vertebrae under complex loading conditions. *Bone.*, 151, 116028. Doi:10.1016/J.Bone.2021.116028.

[19] Leone, A., Cianfoni, A., Zecchi, V., Cortese, M. C., Rumi, N., and Colosimo, C. (2018). Instability and impending instability in patients with vertebral metastatic disease. *Skeletal Radiology.*, Doi:10.1007/S00256-018-3032-3.

[20] Sankey, E. W., Park, C., Howell, E. P., Pennington, Z., Abd-El-Barr, M., Karikari, I. O., … Goodwin, C. R. (2019). Importance of spinal alignment in primary and metastatic spine tumors. *World Neurosurgery.*, Doi:10.1016/J.Wneu.2019.08.161 vc.

[21] Dial, B. L., Catanzano, A. A., Esposito, V., Steele, J., Fletcher, A., Ryan, S. P., Kirkpatrick, J. P., Goodwin, C. R., Torok, J., Hopkins, T., and Mendoza-Lattes, S. (2022). Treatment outcomes in spinal metastatic disease with indeterminate stability. *Global Spine Journal*, 12, 373–380. Doi:10.1177/2192568220956605.

[22] Boussios, S., Cooke, D., Hayward, C., et al. (2018). Metastatic spinal cord compression: Unraveling the diagnostic and therapeutic challenges. *Anticancer Res.*, 38(9), 4987-4997. Doi:10.21873/Anticanres.12817.

[23] Bilsky, Mark H., Ilya, L., Fourney, D. R.; Groff, M., Schmidt, M. H., Varga, P. P., Vrionis, F. D., Yamada, Y., Gerszten, P. C., and Kuklo, T. R. (2010). Reliability analysis of the epidural spinal cord compression scale. *Journal of Neurosurgery: Spine*, 13(3), 324–328. doi:10.3171/2010.3.spine09459.

[24] John, S C., and Roy, A. P. (2008). "Metastatic epidural spinal cord compression." *The Lancet Neurology*, 7.5, 459-466.

[25] Uei, H., MD. Tokuhashi, Y., MD. and Maseda, M. MD. (2018, April 15). Analysis of the relationship between the epidural spinal cord compression (ESCC) scale and paralysis caused by metastatic spine tumors. *SPINE*, 43, Issue 8 pp. E448-E455. DOI: 10.1097/BRS.0000000000002378.

[26] John, S. C., and Roy, A. P. (2008). 'Metastatic epidural spinal cord compression'. *The Lancet Neurology*, 7, no. 5 (May 2008): 459–66. https://doi.org/10.1016/S1474-4422(08)70089-9.

[27] Laufer, I., Sciubba, D. M., Madera, M., et al. (2012). Surgical management of metastatic spinal tumors. *Cancer Control.*, 19(2), 122-128. doi:10.1177/107327 481201900206.

[28] Harel, R., and Angelov, L. (2010). Spine metastases: Current treatments and future directions. *European Journal of Cancer.*, 46(15), 2696-2707. doi:10.1016/j.ejca.201 0.04.025.

[29] Wahood, W., Alexander, A. Y., Yolcu, Y. U., et al. (2021). Trends in utilization of preoperative embolization for spinal metastases: A study of the national inpatient sample 2005–2017. *Neurointervention*, 16(1), 52-58. doi:10.5469/neuroint.2020. 00381.

[30] Hong, S. H., Chang, B. S., Kim, H., Kang, D. H., and Chang, S. Y. (2022). An Updated review on the treatment strategy for spinal metastasis from the spine surgeon's perspective. *Asian Spine Journal*, 16(5), 799–811.

[31] Ilya L., Rubin, D. G., Lis, E., Cox, B. W., Stubblefield, M. D., Yamada, Y., and Bilsky, M. H. (June 2013). *The NOMS Framework: Approach to the Treatment of Spinal Metastatic Tumors, The Oncologist*, 18, Issue 6, pp. 744–751, https://doi.org/ 10.1634/theoncologist.

[32] Joaquim, A. F., Powers, A., Laufer, I., and Bilsky, M. H. (2015). An update in the management of spinal metastases. *Arq Neuro-Psiquiatr.*, 73(9), 795-802. doi:10. 1590/0004-282x20150099.

[33] Patel, D. A., and Campian, J. L. (2017). Diagnostic and therapeutic strategies for patients with malignant epidural spinal cord compression. *Curr. Treat. Options in Oncol.*, 18, 53, https://doi.org/10.1007/s11864-017-0497-6.

[34] Jaipanya, P., Chanplakorn, P. (2022 Apr). Spinal metastasis: narrative reviews of the current evidence and treatment modalities. *J Int Med Res.*, 50(4),

3000605221091665. doi: 10.1177/03000605221091665. PMID: 35437050; PMCID: PMC9021485.

[35] Zeng, K. L., Sahgal, A., Husain, Z. A., Myrehaug, S., Tseng, C. L., Detsky, J., Sarfehnia, A., Ruschin, M., Campbell, M., Foster, M., Das, S., Lipsman, N., Bjarnason, G. A., Atenafu, E. G., Maralani, P. J., Soliman, H. (2021 Mar). Local control and patterns of failure for "Radioresistant" spinal metastases following stereotactic body radiotherapy compared to a "Radiosensitive" reference. *J Neurooncol.*, 152(1), 173-182. doi: 10.1007/s11060-020-03691-6. Epub 2021 Jan 16. PMID: 33453002.

[36] Ivanishvili, Z., and Fourney, D. R. (2014). Incorporating the spine instability neoplastic score into a treatment strategy for spinal metastasis: LMNOP. *Global Spine Journal [Internet]*, 4(2), 129–35. Available from: https://dx.doi.org/10.1055/s-0034-1375560.

[37] Salvo, N., Christakis, M., Rubenstein, J., et al. (2009). The role of plain radiographs in management of bone metastases. *Journal of Palliative Medicine.*, 12(2), 195-198. doi:10.1089/jpm.2008.0055.

[38] Shah, L. M., and Salzman, K. L. (2011). Imaging of spinal metastatic disease. *Int J Surg Oncol.*, 2011, 769753. doi: 10.1155/2011/769753. Epub 2011 Nov 3. PMID: 22312523; PMCID: PMC3263660.

[39] Uchida, K., Nakajima, H., Miyazaki, T., Tsuchida, T., Hirai, T., Sugita, D., Watanabe, S., Takeura, N., Yoshida, A., Okazawa, H., and Baba, H. (2013 Jun). (18)F-FDG PET/CT for diagnosis of osteosclerotic and osteolytic vertebral metastatic lesions: Comparison with bone scintigraphy. *Asian Spine J.*, 7(2), 96-103. doi: 10.4184/asj.2013.7.2.96. Epub 2013 May 22.

[40] Wallace, A. N., Greenwood, T. J., and Jennings, J. W. (2015). Use of imaging in the management of metastatic spine disease with percutaneous ablation and vertebral augmentation. *American Journal of Roentgenology.*, 205(2), 434-441. doi:10.2214/ajr.14.14199.

[41] Polanski, M., and Anderson, N. L. (2006). A list of candidate cancer biomarkers for targeted proteomics. *Biomarker Insights*, 1, 117727190600100.

[42] Peh, W. (2006 Jul). CT-guided percutaneous biopsy of spinal lesions. *Biomed Imaging Interv J.*, 2(3), e25. doi: 10.2349/biij.2.3.e25. Epub 2006 Jul 1. PMID: 21614239; PMCID: PMC3097633.

[43] Ahmad, I., Ahmed, M. M., Ahsraf, M., et al. (September 11, 2018) Pain management in metastatic bone disease: A literature review. *Cureus*, 10(9), e3286. doi:10.7759/cureus.3286

[44] Yakovlev, A. E., and Ellias, Y. (2008). Spinal cord stimulation as a treatment option for intractable neuropathic cancer pain. *Clinical Medicine & Research [Internet]*, 6(3-4), 103–6. Available from: https://dx.doi.org/10.3121/cmr.2008.813.

[45] Porta-Sales, J., Garzón-Rodríguez, C., Llorens-Torromé, S., Brunelli, C., Pigni, A., and Caraceni, A. (2017). Evidence on the analgesic role of bisphosphonates and denosumab in the treatment of pain due to bone metastases: A systematic review within the European Association for Palliative Care guidelines project. *Palliative Medicine.*, 31(1), 5-25. doi:10.1177/0269216316639793.

[46] Kurisunkal, V., Gulia, A., and Gupta, S. (2020). Principles of management of spine metastasis. *JOIO*, 54, 181–193 https://doi.org/10.1007/s43465-019-00008-2.

[47] Ofluoglu, O. (2009). Minimally invasive management of spinal metastases. *Orthopedic Clinics of North America.*, 40(1), 155-168. doi:10.1016/j.ocl.2008.09.006.

[48] Lee, S. K., Weiss, B., Yanamadala, V., Brook, A. (2019). Percutaneous interventional management of spinal metastasis. *Semin Intervent Radiol.*, 36(03), 249-254. doi:10.1055/s-0039-1694698.

[49] Ejima, Y., Matsuo, Y., and Sasaki, R. (2015). The current status future of radiotherapy for spinal bone metastases. *Journal of Orthopedic Science.*, 20(4), 585-592. doi:10.1007/s00776-015-0720-x.

[50] Patchell, R. A., Tibbs, P. A., Regine, W. F., Payne, R., Saris, S., Kryscio, R. J., Mohiuddin, M., and Young, B. (2005). Direct decompressive surgical resection in the treatment of spinal cord compression caused by metastatic cancer: a randomized trial. *Lancet.*, 366(9486), 643–8.

[51] Fisher, (2010). Timing of surgery and radiotherapy in the management of metastatic spine disease: A systematic review. *International Journal of Oncology*, 36., doi:10.3892/ijo_00000527.

[52] Faul, C. M., and Flickinger, J. C. (1995). The use of radiation in the management of spinal metastases. *Journal of Neuro-Oncology*, 23(2), 149–161. doi:10.1007/bf010 53419.10.1007/BF01053419.

[53] Gong, Y., Xu, L., Zhuang, H., Jiang, L., Wei, F., Liu, Z., Li, Y., Yu, M., Ni, K., and Liu, X., (2019). Efficacy and safety of different fractions in stereotactic body radiotherapy for spinal metastases: A systematic review. *Cancer Medicine*, 8, 6176–6184. doi:10.1002/cam4.2546.

[54] Jabbari, S., Gerszten, P. C., Ruschin, M., Larson, D. A., Lo, S. S., and Sahgal, A. (2016). Stereotactic body radiotherapy for spinal metastases. *The Cancer Journal*, 22(4), 280–289. doi:10.1097/ppo.0000000000000205.

[55] Hussain, I., Laufer, I., and Bilsky, M. (2019). Complications of surgery and radiosurgery in spinal metastasis., In *Complications in Neurosurgery*, 356-361. doi:10.1016/b978-0-323-50961-9.00060-8.

[56] Wagner, A., Haag, E., Joerger, A. K., Jost, P., Combs, S. E., Wostrack, M., et al., (2021). Comprehensive surgical treatment strategy for spinal metastases. *Scientific Reports*, 11(1).

[57] Paul K., Jr., and Schmidt, M. H. (2004, April). Surgical management of spinal metastases, *The Oncologist*, 9, Issue 2, pp. 188–196, https://doi.org/10.1634/theonco logist.9-2-188.

[58] Enneking, W. F., Spanier, S. S., Goodman, M. A. (1980 Nov-Dec). A system for the surgical staging of musculoskeletal sarcoma. *Clin Orthop Relat Res.*, (153), 106-20. PMID: 7449206.

[59] Tokuhashi, Y., Uei, H., and Oshima, M. (2017 Dec 20). Classification and scoring systems for metastatic spine tumors: a literature review. *Spine Surg Relat Res.*, 1(2), 44-55. doi: 10.22603/ssrr.1.2016-0021. PMID: 31440612; PMCID: PMC6698555.

[60] Howell, E. P., Williamson, T., Karikari, I., et al. (2019). Total en bloc resection of primary and metastatic spine tumors. *Ann Transl Med.*, 7(10), 226-226. doi:10.2 1037/atm.2019.01.25.

[61] Di Perna, G., Cofano, F., Mantovani, C., Badellino, S., Marengo, N., Ajello, M., Comite, L. M., Palmieri, G., Tartara, F., Zenga, F., Ricardi, U., and Garbossa, D. (2020 Sep). Separation surgery for metastatic epidural spinal cord compression: A qualitative review. *J Bone Oncol.*, 26, 25:100320. doi: 10.1016/j.jbo.2020.100320. PMID: 33088700; PMCID: PMC7559860.

[62] Pennington, Z., Ahmed, A. K., Molina, C. A., Ehresman, J., Laufer, I., and Sciubba, D. M. (2018). Minimally invasive versus conventional spine surgery for vertebral metastases: a systematic review of the evidence. *Annals of Translational Medicine [Internet]*, 6(6), 103–. Available from: https://dx.doi.org/10.21037/atm.2018.01.28.

Chapter 4

The Crucial Role of Estrogen and Relevant Receptors in Cancer Associated Bone Metastasis

Yiran Wang[*]

Department of Obstetrics and Gynecology,
General Hospital of Western Theater Command
of Chinese People's Liberation Army, Chengdu, China

Abstract

Cancer associated metastasis is a unique and special characteristic of malignant tumors during poor progression. Even bone acts as the common tissue to become colonization site due to the tendency of solid tumors, including breast cancer (BCa) and prostate cancer (PCa). Then the osteolytic and osteogenic lesions could be performed during the procedure of bone metastasis. Additionally, bone matrix erosion and regeneration were closely associated with the metabolism of estrogen. In recent years, it has been illustrated that estrogen can play the critical role in affecting the immunological microenvironment of the bone metastasis.

In this chapter, we summarize the impacts of estrogen on immune cells and their consequences on bone homeostasis, metastasis settlement into the bone and relevant poor progression. In addition, the promising application of cancer associated bone metastasis is also discussed by targeting estrogen and its associated receptors.

Keywords: estrogen, estrogen receptors, bone marrow, micro-environment, immunological balance, bone metastasis

---

[*] Corresponding Author's Email: yiranwang1993@sina.com.

In: New Research on Bone Metastasis
Editor: Joseph Gerfried
ISBN: 979-8-88697-799-8
© 2023 Nova Science Publishers, Inc.

Introduction

Estrogen acts as a kind of steroid hormone, which contains estradiol, estrone, estriol, and estetrol. In addition, it is known to us that it could be synthesized and released from mammalian ovaries and participates in regulating the differentiation or development of sexual organs and maintaining the dynamic balance of the reproductive system [1-2]. Moreover, estrogen exhibits its various physiological functions in the immunological system, musculoskeletal system, and so on [3]. In particular, estrogens are the main partners in both skeletal growth and skeletal maintenance, including normal bone mineral density and trabecular bone mass during adult life. Moreover, reduced levels of estrogen can be related to the poor progression of osteoporosis and cancer-associated bone metastasis [4-5]. In this chapter, we have drawn our eyes on the modulatory roles of estrogen as well as estrogen-related receptors in cancer-associated bone metastasis.

In the pathophysiological station, estrogens display their relevant biological functions through direct and indirect regulatory signaling pathways. Upon estrogens make binding to two nuclear receptor subtypes such as estrogen receptor-a (ERa) and ER-β, these signaling cascades could be activated. While the ligand functional points are occupied, they could translocate to the nucleus and make function as transcription factors by binding to dedicated DNA sequences [6]. In this regard, ERa can activate and induce the MAPK signaling cascade by modulating the phosphorylation MEK, ERK, and JNK via making the coupling effects with transcriptional factors such as c-jun and Elk-1 [7]. When the ERs bind with ligand, the ligand-bound ERs can bind to ER elements in the genome and stimulate structural changes of chromatin to recruit coactivators and factors [8]. In addition, three orphan nuclear receptors referred to as Estrogen Receptor-Related Receptors (ERRs) ERRa, ERRb and ERRg have been described [9]. Moreover, several research has shown that ERRa participates in bone matrix metabolism by targeting the estrogen signaling pathway [10-12].

Bone metastasis is a common complication of many cancers, of which prostate cancer (PCa) and breast cancer (BCa) are the most common, with an incidence of 73% and 68% individually [13]. The development of bone metastasis requires that cancer cells exudate and homing to bone marrow through interaction with endothelial cells, osteoblasts, osteoclasts, and any other cells in the micro-environment. Once cancer cells migrate to the bone, the cancer cells will disrupt the dynamic balance of bone resorption and bone formation. In addition to bone marrow-derived cells, several kinds of immunological cells in bone marrow (BM) also strongly affect the procedure of bone metastasis [13]. Interestingly, estrogen deficiency is the most common cause for bone metastasis because sex steroids associated with estrogen deficiency and reduced inflammatory tension to alter the bone microenvironment, mainly osteoclasts, thus stimulating the anchoring, survival, and osteolytic phenotype of cancer cells [14].

In contrast, in several clinical studies, the incidence of bone marrow disseminated tumor cells (DTC) in premenopausal women (32.7%) was slightly higher than that in postmenopausal women (29.5%), indicating that postmenopausal women acquired lower risk of bone metastasis [15]. It is worth noting that all immune cells present in bones are also highly expressed with ER [16], and there is growing evidence that estrogen plays a role in bone metastasis through making complex effects with any other immunological cells.

The purpose of this chapter is to introduce existing knowledge and our ideas on the relationship between estrogen signals in osteoimmunological micro-environment and their effects on the homing and progression of metastatic cells in the bone marrow.

Estrogen in Osteoclasts

Osteoclasts are also derived from mononuclear / macrophage lines. However, under inflammatory conditions, osteoclasts can come from either dendritic cells or hematopoietic progenitor cells [17-19]. In addition to the indirect effects of estrogen on osteoclast differentiation, it has been reported that selective removal of Era from osteoclasts can lead to a trabecular loss in female mice by reducing FasL expression and autocrine regulation, thus inhibiting osteoclast apoptosis. As for macrophages/monocytes, osteoclasts are also antigen-presenting cells that activate CD4+T and CD8+T cells and are endowed with the unique ability to stimulate Foxp3+ regulatory T cells (Treg) [20-21]. In addition, osteoclasts produce many chemokines (CCL13, CCL14, CCL5, CXCL5, CCL10, CXCL11) that attract a variety of immune cells, such as monocytes, macrophages, T cells, NK cells, and DC cells [22].

PCA-derived BMET activates osteoclast formation by producing nuclear factor Kappa-B receptor activator ligand (RANKL) in osteoblasts, thereby increasing the function of osteoblasts and promoting their growth in bone [23]. ERRα is also a powerful regulator of osteoclast differentiation [24-25]. Interestingly, depending on the source of metastasis, the overexpression of

ERRα in cancer cells may inhibit or stimulate osteoclasts by stimulating the expression of OPG (osteoprotegerin), which is the main inhibitor of osteoclast activity in cells, or the expression of VEGF-A and WNT5A in PCa cells.

At present, the effect of estrogen on ERRα in tumor and their role in the regulation of BMET remain to be determined. Through its action on osteoclasts, estrogen inhibits bone resorption but also changes the ability of osteoclasts to interact and recruit other immune cells to the bone, directly affecting the development of pro-inflammatory microenvironment conducive to bone metastasis (Figure 1).

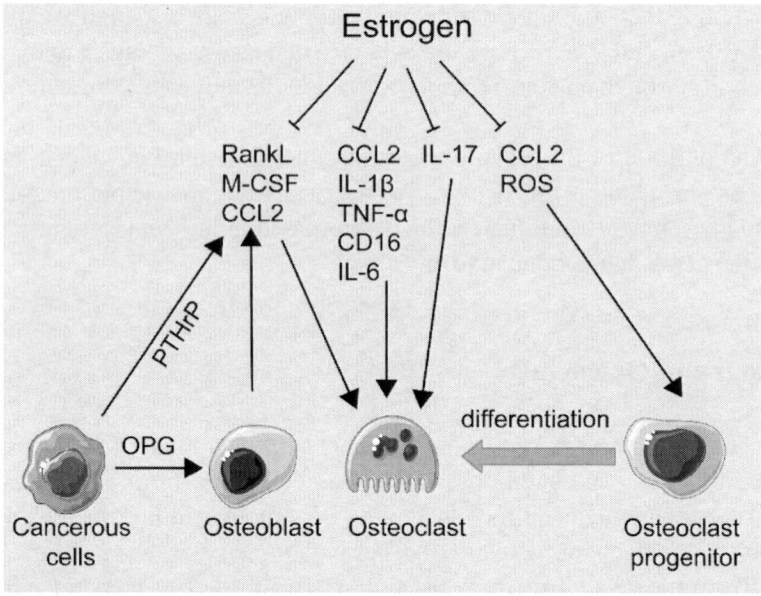

Figure 1. The close correlation among the estrogen in the bone metastasis during immunological micro-environment.

Estrogen in Monocytes-Macrophages

In addition to neutropenia, estrogen inhibits the differentiation of mononuclear phagocytes. In fact, estrogen reduces the levels of macrophage colony-stimulating factor (M-CSF) and granulocyte-macrophage colony-stimulating factor (GM-CSF). M-CSF is mainly produced by osteocytes, osteoblasts, and osteoblast precursors. Granulocyte-macrophage colony-stimulating factor (GM-CSF) is mainly secreted by a variety of cells in bone, mainly in response to dangerous stimuli [26-28]. Bone marrow-derived macrophages are mostly produced by the differentiation of monocytes back into the bone. In addition to inhibiting the differentiation of monocytes/macrophages, estrogen also reduces the concentration of CCL2 produced by osteoblasts and osteocytes, thereby reducing the recruitment of monocytes and macrophage precursors expressing CCR2 to bone [29]. Estrogen also directly inhibits the production of CCL2 by monocytes/macrophages, thus inhibiting the recruitment from bone [30].

Interestingly, estrogen has different direct effects on monocyte/macrophage function depending on the endoplasmic reticulum signaling. In monocytes/macrophages, E2/ERα has been shown to reduce osteoclast differentiation by inhibiting the production of pro-inflammatory cytokines, such as IL-1β, TNF-α, and IL-6. On the contrary, E2/ERβ inhibits the expression of CD16 at the cell surface, thus inhibiting the procedure of ADCC (antigen-dependent cytotoxicity) [31]. Whether the different stages of macrophage maturation are more closely related to the expression of one type of ER than another type of ER remains to be solved.

The expression of ERRα in several tissues, including bone, is up-regulated by modulated with estrogen [32] and participates in the making function with macrophages. Additionally, it can regulate the response of macrophages to TLR4 and the production of ROS [33]. Through their strong phagocytic activity, macrophages represent powerful cells that can eliminate metastatic cells that reach the bone, although they can also affect BMET through other mechanisms that can be targeted by estrogen. Indeed, estrogen strongly affects macrophage polarization and transition of subtypes by promoting M2 (promoting osteoblasts) polarization and inhibiting M1 (promoting osteoclasts) polarization [34]. Therefore, by promoting M1 macrophages, estrogen deficiency inhibits M2 production of BMP2 and stimulates M1 production of ROS, nitric oxide, and pro-inflammatory cytokines, thereby promoting bone resorption [35].

It is noted that the dynamic balance of M2 macrophages is useful to establish the suitable micro-environment for bone metastasis through promoting metastatic angiogenesis and tumor invasion by producing VEGF-A in the micro-environment [36]. In bones, a special subgroup of macrophages, called bone macrophages has been described. Bone macrophages (TRAP-F4/80+, CD68+, Mac3+) exist on the bone surface near osteoblasts and support osteogenic function and bone matrix metabolism [37]. The data show that the level of estrogen is related to the function of bone macrophages because the number of bone macrophages in trabecular and cortical bone increases after ovariectomy. Interestingly, in this case, bone macrophages contain intracellular vesicles in TRAP+ cells, which demonstrates their "cleaning" effect on excreted absorptive vesicles released by osteoclasts (TRAP+) [38]. BMET derived from PCa increases the function of osteoblasts through the CCL2 [39]. Tumor-associated macrophages (TAM) can enhance the BMET of BCa and PCa. An increase in the number of CD206+M2-like macrophages was also found in PCa BMET. The expression of CCL2 in cancer cells promotes the recruitment of TAM expressing CCR2 to promote the anchoring of cancer cells in bone [40]. Similarly, the expression of parathyroid hormone-associated protein (PTHrP) in BCa and PCa cells upregulates CCL2 production in osteoblasts, which contributes to macrophage recruitment to bone, bone remodeling, and BMET progression [41].

In addition, phagocytosis of tumor apoptotic cells can promote the production of CXCL5 by macrophages and promote the inflammatory bone microenvironment that supports BMET development [42]. Therefore, estrogen inhibits the number of monocytes/macrophages in bones, including bone macrophages, and affects their function. Estrogen enhances the production of non-inflammatory cytokines, inhibits bone remodeling, and prevents the formation of fertile soil anchored by BMET. However, once BMET manages to stabilize in bone, estrogen provides a microenvironment that promotes tumor progression by acting on macrophages (Figure 1).

Estrogen in Bone Homeostasis during Bone Metastasis

T cells and T lymphocytes present in bone marrow account for less than 5% of CD45+ cells, and the CD4/CD8 ratio is lower than that in blood [43]. A large number of T cells in BM are memory cells, which either circulate or permanently reside in BM, indicating that BM T cells can form T cell pools specific to antigens exposed to cancer cells in the context of BMET [44]. T cells entering the bone marrow are largely supported by CXCL12 produced by osteoblasts and stromal cells and down-regulated by estrogen [45]. In the absence of *in vivo / in situ* labeling data, so far there is no direct evidence that estrogen affects T cell retention in bone. However, this phenomenon is largely determined by the interaction between integrin-$\alpha 4\beta 1$ on the surface of T cells and VCAM-1 expressed by stromal cells and endothelial cells, and is described as down-regulated by estrogen [46-47].

One of the main effects of estrogen on bone marrow T cells is to inhibit their osteoclast differentiation. Evidence of this function appeared more than

20 years ago, when it was observed that nude mice were not affected by trabecular loss caused by ovariectomy compared with wild-type mice. Later, CD4+T cells that produce IL-17 and RANKL in bones were identified as effective osteoclast-producing stimuli [48]. Th17 cells are suggested to establish a pre-bone metastasis niche, which helps cancer cells to implant into the bone [49]. In addition, Th17 cells are recommended to rule out BMET-controlled anti-PD1 therapy [50]. Estrogen directly controls the Th17 cell pool because ERA binds to the RORC promoter that suppresses the expression of ROR-γ T cells.

In addition to Th17 cell differentiation, estrogen also inhibits Th1 cell programming [51]. In bone marrow, estrogen deficiency impairs the production of transforming growth factor-β by stromal cells, a cytokine that plays a key role in inhibiting the expression of T-Bet and interferon-γ / tumor necrosis factor-α in T cells [52] and thus plays a key role in osteoclast formation [53]. Considering the strong role of transforming growth factor-b in inhibiting the expression of granzyme A,-B and FasL in CD8+T cells [54], the ability of estrogen to maintain the level of transforming growth factor-b in bone marrow weakens the cytotoxic function of CD8+T cells and promotes the progression of bone marrow interstitial fibrosis [55]. However, the control of estrogen / estrogen signal on the level of transforming growth factor-β in bone and BMET is more complex. In fact, bones contain a large amount of transforming growth factor-β, which is stored in its mineralized matrix and is released and activated by osteoclasts.

Additionally, BMET also helps to increase the level of transforming growth factor-b [56]. ERR-alpha is also obviously involved in the activation of effector T cells [57]. In BCa BMET, the expression of ERR-alpha inhibits the production of transforming growth factor-b by cancer cells, intensifies the cytotoxicity of CD8+T cells in bone, and effectively controls BMET [58]. Transforming growth factor-β is associated with increased production and stability of Tregs [59]. In bone marrow, the proportion of Tregs in CD4+T cells is much higher than that in lymph nodes, which may be due to the high expression of CXCR4 on Tregs, which is largely promoted by estrogen [60]. Once the cancer cells are anchored, Treg produces large amounts of RANKL, which promotes osteolysis associated with the feedback cycle of transforming growth factor-b release in BCA BMET [61]. Thus, in bones, the effect of estrogen on T cells is twofold: by promoting an immunosuppressive environment associated with decreased activity of CD8+T cells and an increase in the number of Tregs that promotes tumor growth, and by inhibiting RANKL production by Th1 and Th17 cells to limit osteolysis (Figure 1).

Conclusion and Perspective

Recently, as is known to us that estrogen could closely participate in modulating bone homeostasis by making coupling effects with any other immunological cells. Then, it is noted that adult women could acquire stronger immune responses than men via innate and acquired immune responses during aging. Subsequently, administration with estrogen may have an indirectly anti-tumor effects by regulating the dynamic balance of immune system, which may be involved in the regulation of pre-metastatic niche and/or the tumor associated immunological environment in bone. Then, it is valuable to develop more and more effective treatment strategies for cancer associated bone metastasis by targeting estrogen and relevant receptors.

References

[1] Xu X L, Huang Z Y, Yu K, Li J, Fu X W, Deng S L. Estrogen Biosynthesis and Signal Transduction in Ovarian Disease. *Front. Endocrinol. (Lausanne).* 2022;13: 827032. Published 2022 Mar 1. doi:10.3389/fendo.2022.827032.
[2] Hilton H N, Clarke C L, Graham J D. Estrogen and progesterone signalling in the normal breast and its implications for cancer development. *Mol. Cell Endocrinol.* 2018;466:2-14. doi:10.1016/j.mce.2017.08.011.
[3] De Paoli M, Zakharia A, Werstuck G H. The Role of Estrogen in Insulin Resistance: A Review of Clinical and Preclinical Data. *Am. J. Pathol.* 2021;191(9):1490-1498. doi:10.1016/j.ajpath.2021.05.011.
[4] Fischer A, Bardakci F, Sellner M, Lill M A, Smieško M. Ligand pathways in estrogen-related receptors. *J. Biomol. Struct. Dyn.* 2023;41(5):1639-1648. doi:10. 1080/07391102.2022.2027818.
[5] Shropshire D B, Acosta F M, Fang K, Benavides J, Sun L-Z, Jin V X & Jiang J X. Association of adenosine signaling gene signature with estrogen receptor-positive breast and prostate cancer bone metastasis. *Front. Med. (Lausanne).* 2022;9:965429. Published 2022 Sep 15. doi:10.3389/fmed.2022.965429.
[6] Chakraborty B, Byemerwa J, Krebs T, Lim F, Chang C Y, McDonnell D P. Estrogen Receptor Signaling in the Immune System. *Endocr. Rev.* 2023;44(1):117-141. doi:10.1210/endrev/bnac017.
[7] Mahboobifard F, Pourgholami M H, Jorjani M, Dargahi L, Amiri M, Sadeghi S & Tehrani F R. Estrogen as a key regulator of energy homeostasis and metabolic health. *Biomed. Pharmacother.* 2022;156:113808. doi:10.1016/j.biopha.2022.1138 08.
[8] Yoh K, Ikeda K, Horie K, Inoue S. Roles of Estrogen, Estrogen Receptors, and Estrogen-Related Receptors in Skeletal Muscle: Regulation of Mitochondrial

Function. *Int. J. Mol. Sci.* 2023;24(3):1853. Published 2023 Jan 17. doi:10.3390/ijms24031853.

[9] Tecalco-Cruz A C, López-Canovas L, Azuara-Liceaga E. Estrogen signaling via estrogen receptor alpha and its implications for neurodegeneration associated with Alzheimer's disease in aging women [published online ahead of print, 2023 Jan 14]. *Metab. Brain Dis.* 2023;10.1007/s11011-023-01161-2. doi:10.1007/s11011-023-01161-2.

[10] Maitra R, Malik P, Mukherjee T K. Targeting Estrogens and Various Estrogen-Related Receptors against Non-Small Cell Lung Cancers: A Perspective. *Cancers (Basel).* 2021;14(1):80. Published 2021 Dec 24. doi:10.3390/cancers14010080.

[11] Tang J, Liu T, Wen X, Zhou Z, Yan J, Gao J & Zuo J. Estrogen-related receptors: novel potential regulators of osteoarthritis pathogenesis. *Mol. Med.* 2021;27(1):5. Published 2021 Jan 15. doi:10.1186/s10020-021-00270-x.

[12] Crevet L, Vanacker J M. Regulation of the expression of the estrogen related receptors (ERRs). *Cell Mol. Life Sci.* 2020;77(22):4573-4579. doi:10.1007/s00018-020-03549-0.

[13] Song M K, Park S I, Cho S W. Circulating biomarkers for diagnosis and therapeutic monitoring in bone metastasis [published online ahead of print, 2023 Feb 2]. *J. Bone Miner. Metab.* 2023;10.1007/s00774-022-01396-6. doi:10.1007/s00774-022-01396-6.

[14] Browne A J, Kubasch M L, Göbel A, Hadji P, Chen D, Rauner M, Stölzel F, Hofbauer L C & Rachner T D. Concurrent antitumor and bone-protective effects of everolimus in osteotropic breast cancer. *Breast Cancer Res.* 2017;19(1):92. Published 2017 Aug 9. doi:10.1186/s13058-017-0885-7.

[15] Tian Y, Riquelme M A, Tu C, Quan Y, Liu X, Sun L-Z & Jiang J X. Osteocytic Connexin Hemichannels Modulate Oxidative Bone Microenvironment and Breast Cancer Growth. *Cancers (Basel).* 2021;13(24):6343. Published 2021 Dec 17. doi:10.3390/cancers13246343.

[16] Ihle C L, Wright-Hobart S J, Owens P. Therapeutics targeting the metastatic breast cancer bone microenvironment. *Pharmacol. Ther.* 2022;239:108280. doi:10.1016/j.pharmthera.2022.108280.

[17] Veis D J, O'Brien C A. Osteoclasts, Master Sculptors of Bone. *Annu. Rev. Pathol.* 2023;18:257-281. doi:10.1146/annurev-pathmechdis-031521-040919.

[18] Weivoda M M, Bradley E W. Macrophages and Bone Remodeling [published online ahead of print, 2023 Jan 18]. *J. Bone Miner. Res.* 2023;10.1002/jbmr.4773. doi:10.1002/jbmr.4773.

[19] Srivastava R K, Sapra L, Mishra P K. Osteometabolism: Metabolic Alterations in Bone Pathologies. *Cells.* 2022;11(23):3943. Published 2022 Dec 6. doi:10.3390/cells11233943.

[20] Okamoto K, Takayanagi H. Effect of T cells on bone. *Bone.* 2023;168:116675. doi:10.1016/j.bone.2023.116675.

[21] Zuo H, Wan Y. Inhibition of myeloid PD-L1 suppresses osteoclastogenesis and cancer bone metastasis. *Cancer Gene Ther.* 2022;29(10):1342-1354. doi:10.1038/s41417-022-00446-5.

[22] Okamoto K, Takayanagi H. Osteoimmunology. *Cold Spring Harb. Perspect Med.* 2019;9(1):a031245. Published 2019 Jan 2. doi:10.1101/cshperspect.a031245.

[23] Takayanagi H. Osteoimmunology - Bidirectional dialogue and inevitable union of the fields of bone and immunity. *Proc. Jpn. Acad. Ser. B Phys. Biol. Sci.* 2020;96(4):159-169. doi:10.2183/pjab.96.013.

[24] Feng C, Xu Z, Tang X, Cao H, Zhang G, Tan J. Estrogen-Related Receptor α: A Significant Regulator and Promising Target in Bone Homeostasis and Bone Metastasis. *Molecules.* 2022;27(13):3976. Published 2022 Jun 21. doi:10.3390/molecules27133976.

[25] Carnesecchi J, Vanacker J M. Estrogen-Related Receptors and the control of bone cell fate. *Mol. Cell Endocrinol.* 2016;432:37-43. doi:10.1016/j.mce.2015.07.019.

[26] Atanga E, Dolder S, Dauwalder T, Wetterwald A, Hofstetter W. TNFα inhibits the development of osteoclasts through osteoblast-derived GM-CSF. *Bone.* 2011;49(5):1090-1100. doi:10.1016/j.bone.2011.08.003.

[27] Ruef N, Dolder S, Aeberli D, Seitz M, Balani D, Hofstetter W. Granulocyte-macrophage colony-stimulating factor-dependent CD11c-positive cells differentiate into active osteoclasts. *Bone.* 2017;97:267-277. doi:10.1016/j.bone.2017.01.036.

[28] Postiglione L, Domenico G D, Montagnani S, Spigna G D, Salzano S, Castaldo C, Ramaglia L, Sbordone L & Rossi G. Granulocyte-macrophage colony-stimulating factor (GM-CSF) induces the osteoblastic differentiation of the human osteosarcoma cell line SaOS-2. *Calcif. Tissue Int.* 2003;72(1):85-97. doi:10.1007/s00223-001-2088-5.

[29] Biguetti C C, Vieira A E, Cavalla F, Fonseca A C, Colavite P M, Silva R M, Trombone A P F & Garlet G P. CCR2 Contributes to F4/80+ Cells Migration Along Intramembranous Bone Healing in Maxilla, but Its Deficiency Does Not Critically Affect the Healing Outcome. *Front. Immunol.* 2018;9:1804. Published 2018 Aug 10. doi:10.3389/fimmu.2018.01804.

[30] Yang X W, Wang X S, Cheng F B, Wang F, Wan L, Wang F & Huang H-X. Elevated CCL2/MCP-1 Levels are Related to Disease Severity in Postmenopausal Osteoporotic Patients. *Clin. Lab.* 2016;62(11):2173-2181. doi:10.7754/Clin.Lab.2016.160408.

[31] Song T, Lin T, Ma J, Guo L, Zhang L, Zhou X & Ye T. Regulation of TRPV5 transcription and expression by E2/ERα signalling contributes to inhibition of osteoclastogenesis. *J. Cell Mol. Med.* 2018;22(10):4738-4750. doi:10.1111/jcmm.13718.

[32] Giguère V. To ERR in the estrogen pathway. *Trends Endocrinol Metab.* 2002;13(5):220-225. doi:10.1016/s1043-2760(02)00592-1.

[33] Guo P, Xu J, Liang H, Xu L, Gao W, Chen Z, Gao Y, Zhang M, Yu G & Shao Z. Estrogen Suppresses Cytokines Release in cc4821 *Neisseria meningitidis* Infection via TLR4 and ERβ-p38-MAPK Pathway. *Front. Microbiol.* 2022;13:834091. Published 2022 Mar 29. doi:10.3389/fmicb.2022.834091.

[34] Yin J J, Pollock C B, Kelly K. Mechanisms of cancer metastasis to the bone. *Cell Res.* 2005;15(1):57-62. doi:10.1038/sj.cr.7290266.

[35] Khosla S, Oursler M J, Monroe D G. Estrogen and the skeleton. *Trends Endocrinol Metab.* 2012;23(11):576-581. doi:10.1016/j.tem.2012.03.008.

[36] Ge Y W, Liu X L, Yu D G, Zhu Z A, Ke Q F, Mao Y Q, Guo Y P & Zhang J W. Graphene-modified CePO4 nanorods effectively treat breast cancer-induced bone metastases and regulate macrophage polarization to improve osteo-inductive ability [published correction appears in *J. Nanobiotechnology*. 2021 Mar 30;19(1):91]. *J. Nanobiotechnology*. 2021;19(1):11. Published 2021 Jan 7. doi:10.1186/s12951-020-00753-9.

[37] Yao Y, Cai X, Ren F, Ye Y, Wang F, Zheng C, Qian Y & Zhang M. The Macrophage-Osteoclast Axis in Osteoimmunity and Osteo-Related Diseases. *Front. Immunol.* 2021;12:664871. Published 2021 Mar 31. doi:10.3389/fimmu.2021.664871.

[38] Yang D, Wan Y. Molecular determinants for the polarization of macrophage and osteoclast. *Semin. Immunopathol.* 2019;41(5):551-563. doi:10.1007/s00281-019-00754-3.

[39] Siddiqui J A, Seshacharyulu P, Muniyan S, Pothuraju R, Khan P, Vengoji R, Chaudhary S, Maurya S K, Lele S M, Jain M, Datta K, Nasser M W & Batra S K. GDF15 promotes prostate cancer bone metastasis and colonization through osteoblastic CCL2 and RANKL activation. *Bone Res.* 2022;10(1):6. Published 2022 Jan 20. doi:10.1038/s41413-021-00178-6.

[40] Misawa A, Kondo Y, Takei H, Takizawa T. Long Noncoding RNA *HOXA11-AS* and Transcription Factor HOXB13 Modulate the Expression of Bone Metastasis-Related Genes in Prostate Cancer. *Genes (Basel)*. 2021;12(2):182. Published 2021 Jan 27. doi:10.3390/genes12020182.

[41] Lee G T, Kwon S J, Kim J, Kwon Y S, Lee N, Hong J H, Jamieson C, Kim W-J & Kim I Y. WNT5A induces castration-resistant prostate cancer via CCL2 and tumor-infiltrating macrophages. *Br. J. Cancer.* 2018;118(5):670-678. doi:10.1038/bjc.2017.451.

[42] Roca H, Jones J D, Purica M C, Weidner S, Koh A J, Kuo R, Wilkinson J E, Wang Y, Daignault-Newton S, Pienta K J, Morgan T M, Keller E T, Nör J E, Shea L D & McCauley L K. Apoptosis-induced CXCL5 accelerates inflammation and growth of prostate tumor metastases in bone. *J. Clin. Invest.* 2018;128(1):248-266. doi:10.1172/JCI92466.

[43] Crespo J, Sun H, Welling T H, Tian Z, Zou W. T cell anergy, exhaustion, senescence, and stemness in the tumor microenvironment. *Curr. Opin. Immunol.* 2013;25(2):214-221. doi:10.1016/j.coi.2012.12.003.

[44] Kfoury Y, Baryawno N, Severe N, Mei S, Gustafsson K, Hirz T, Brouse T, Scadden E W, Igolkina A A, Kokkaliaris K, Choi B D, Barkas N, Randolph M A, Shin J H, Saylor P J, Scadden D T, Sykes D B & Kharchenko P V. Human prostate cancer bone metastases have an actionable immunosuppressive microenvironment. *Cancer Cell.* 2021;39 (11):1464-1478.e8. doi:10.1016/j.ccell.2021.09.005.

[45] Ponte F, Kim H N, Iyer S, Han L, Almeida M, Manolagas S C. Cxcl12 Deletion in Mesenchymal Cells Increases Bone Turnover and Attenuates the Loss of Cortical Bone Caused by Estrogen Deficiency in Mice. *J. Bone Miner. Res.* 2020;35(8):1441-1451. doi:10.1002/jbmr.4002.

[46] Iida J, Meijne A M, Spiro R C, Roos E, Furcht L T, McCarthy J B. Spreading and focal contact formation of human melanoma cells in response to the stimulation of

both melanoma-associated proteoglycan (NG2) and alpha 4 beta 1 integrin. *Cancer Res.* 1995;55(10):2177-2185.

[47] Yao W, Guan M, Jia J, Dai W, Lay Y-A. E, Amugongo S, Liu R, Olivos D, Saunders M, Lam K S, Nolta J, Olvera D, Ritchie R O & Lane N E. Reversing bone loss by directing mesenchymal stem cells to bone [published correction appears in Stem Cells. 2014 Feb;32(2):601]. *Stem Cells.* 2013;31(9):2003-2014. doi:10.1002/stem.1461.

[48] Ibáñez L, Abou-Ezzi G, Ciucci T, Amiot V, Belaïd N, Obino D, Mansour A, Rouleau M, Wakkach A & Blin-Wakkach C. Inflammatory Osteoclasts Prime TNFα-Producing CD4$^+$ T Cells and Express CX$_3$CR1. *J. Bone Miner Res.* 2016; 31(10):1899-1908. doi:10.1002/jbmr.2868.

[49] Monteiro A C, Bonomo A. CD8$^+$ T cells from experimental *in situ* breast carcinoma interfere with bone homeostasis. *Bone.* 2021;150:116014. doi:10.1016/j.bone.2021.116014.

[50] Wang K, Gu Y, Liao Y, Bang S, Donnelly C R, Chen O, Tao X, Mirando A J, Hilton M J & Ji R-R. PD-1 blockade inhibits osteoclast formation and murine bone cancer pain. *J. Clin. Invest.* 2020;130(7):3603-3620. doi:10.1172/JCI133334.

[51] Salem M L. Estrogen, a double-edged sword: modulation of TH1- and TH2-mediated inflammations by differential regulation of TH1/TH2 cytokine production. *Curr. Drug Targets Inflamm. Allergy.* 2004;3(1):97-104. doi:10.2174/1568010043483944.

[52] Cenci S, Toraldo G, Weitzmann M N, Roggia C, Gao Y, Qian W P, Sierra O & Pacifici R. Estrogen deficiency induces bone loss by increasing T cell proliferation and lifespan through IFN-gamma-induced class II transactivator. *Proc. Natl. Acad. Sci. USA.* 2003;100(18):10405-10410. doi:10.1073/pnas.1533207100.

[53] Tsukasaki M, Takayanagi H. Osteoimmunology: evolving concepts in bone-immune interactions in health and disease. *Nat. Rev. Immunol.* 2019;19(10):626-642. doi:10.1038/s41577-019-0178-8.

[54] Mishra S, Srinivasan S, Ma C, Zhang N. CD8$^+$ Regulatory T Cell - A Mystery to Be Revealed. *Front. Immunol.* 2021;12:708874. Published 2021 Aug 18. doi:10.3389/fimmu.2021.708874.

[55] Kowalczyk K, Franik G, Kowalczyk D, Pluta D, Blukacz Ł, Madej P. Thyroid disorders in polycystic ovary syndrome. *Eur. Rev. Med. Pharmacol. Sci.* 2017;21(2): 346-360.

[56] Shah A H, Tabayoyong W B, Kundu S D, Kim S-J, Van Parijs L, Liu V C, Kwon E, Greenberg N M, Lee C. Suppression of tumor metastasis by blockade of transforming growth factor beta signaling in bone marrow cells through a retroviral-mediated gene therapy in mice. *Cancer Res.* 2002;62(24):7135-7138.

[57] Shu C, Wang C, Chen S, Huang X, Cui J, Li W & Xu B. ERR-activated GPR35 promotes immune infiltration level of macrophages in gastric cancer tissues. *Cell Death Discov.* 2022;8(1):444. Published 2022 Nov 4. doi:10.1038/s41420-022-01238-4.

[58] Yoon T J, Koppula S, Lee K H. The effects of β-glucans on cancer metastasis. *Anticancer Agents Med. Chem.* 2013;13(5):699-708. doi:10.2174/18715206113130 50004.

[59] Kimura A, Kishimoto T. IL-6: regulator of Treg/Th17 balance. *Eur. J. Immunol.* 2010; 40(7):1830-1835. doi:10.1002/eji.201040391.
[60] Fan X L, Duan X B, Chen Z H, Li M, Xu J S, Ding G M. Lack of estrogen down-regulates CXCR4 expression on Treg cells and reduces Treg cell population in bone marrow in OVX mice. *Cell Mol. Biol. (Noisy-le-grand).* 2015;61(2):13-17. Published 2015 May 8.
[61] Karavitis J, Hix L M, Shi Y H, Schultz R F, Khazaie K, Zhang M. Regulation of COX2 expression in mouse mammary tumor cells controls bone metastasis and PGE2-induction of regulatory T cell migration. *PLoS One.* 2012;7(9):e46342. doi:10.1371/journal.pone.0046342.

Chapter 5

Evolving Cancer–Bone Coupling Effects During Bone Metastasis

Fangze Xing[1]
Hui Qiang[2],*
and Pei Yang[1]

[1] Department of Bone and Joint Surgery,
The Second Affiliated Hospital of Xi'an Jiaotong University,
Xi'an, People's Republic of China
[2] Department of Orthopaedic Surgery,
The Third Affiliated Hospital of Xi'an Jiaotong University,
Xi'an, People's Republic of China

Abstract

Uncontrolled development, invasion, and metastasis are characteristics of cancer, the leading cause of death among patients worldwide. After the lung and liver, the bone marrow is the third most typical location for tumor spread. Tumor cells can escape with the primary tumor site, be customized to the bone microenvironment, and use the bone as a launch pad for further metastasis to other organs. As the tumor cells travel from the primary focus to the bone, they establish interactions with the bone microenvironment, and these interactions determine the fate of the cancer cells.

Bone is a highly dynamic tissue whose dynamic balance is coordinated by osteoclasts that destroy bone, osteoblasts that form bone, and mechanosensory osteoclasts. The interaction of hormones, paracrine growth factors, and cytokines also regulates this dynamic process. As a

---

* Coresponding Author's Email: E-mail: qianghui359@163.com.

In: New Research on Bone Metastasis
Editor: Joseph Gerfried
ISBN: 979-8-88697-799-8
© 2023 Nova Science Publishers, Inc.

person ages, catabolism predominates in bone metabolism, and year-on-year bone loss reduces the strength of the bone while weakening its ability to repair damage caused by malignant infiltrative disease. The bone marrow can act as a remote responder for tumors at the primary focus and as a source of cells that recruit other organs to form premetastatic niche formation. Most tumor cells that leave the primary site are destroyed before they can establish metastasis. However, a small proportion of the surviving tumor cells are attracted by chemotaxis to the 'metastatic niche' in the hematopoietic bone marrow.

The first niche of disseminated tumor cells (DTC) in the bone microenvironment plays an essential role in subsequent metastasis. Tumor cells can induce osteoblasts to secrete RANKL by secreting osteolytic factors, which regulate osteoclastogenesis. Resorption of the bone matrix by over-activated osteoclasts leads to the release of numerous cytokines, which further act on the cancer cells to form an osteolytic vicious cycle. This process causes events such as bone marrow compression and pathological fractures. The asymptomatic phase of bone colonization may last for several years and is characterized by resting disseminated tumor cells with proliferating bone micrometastases, based on which the elimination of the tumourigenic capacity of DTC and BMM can effectively eliminate dormant cancer cells. The metastasis-limiting interactions of tumor cells with various cellular and non-cellular components of the bone marrow niche provide precious therapeutic targets.

Introduction

Bone is a dynamic tissue that remodels continuously throughout life, provides mechanical support for height and movement, and is also a reservoir of calcium and phosphate (Kim et al., 2020). Uncontrolled development, invasion, and metastasis are characteristics of cancer, the leading cause of death among patients worldwide. After the lung and liver, the bone marrow is the third most typical location for tumor spread (Clarke 2008; Rodan 1998).

Metastasis is the leading cause of death from cancer, and bone is the third most common site of metastasis after lung and liver (Mundy 2002; Weilbaecher, Guise, and McCauley 2011; Kingsley et al., 2007). Breast cancer and prostate cancer are common in women and men, respectively, and although most solid tumors can be removed surgically, over 90% of patients die from metastases (Gupta and Massagué 2006). However, there is a paucity of treatments for metastases, particularly bone metastases.

Cancer cells from the initial tumor must first go through epithelial-to-mesenchymal transition (EMT) in order to invade nearby tissues and get into the blood or lymphatic system, where they then move to distant organs and establish themselves in that microenvironment (Chaffer et al., 2016; Puisieux, Brabletz, and Caramel 2014). The period between primary tumor diagnosis and metastasis is called metastatic dormancy, during which disseminated tumor cells (DTC) survive and subsequently form large secondary tumors (metastases). Although metastases are a very inefficient process, once they are formed, they are responsible for 90% of cancer-related mortality. The ability to target DTC and micrometastases to adapt and colonise secondary loci may be a viable approach to eliminating metastases (Kang and Pantel 2013; Muscarella et al., 2021; Pantel, Brakenhoff, and Brandt 2008). So, in order to research therapeutic strategies that could enhance patient prognosis, it is crucial to further understand the cellular and molecular pathways linked to metastasis formation.

The complex and protracted process of bone metastasis involves the invasion of tumor cells into the bone marrow, adaptation to the microenvironment, the creation of cancer niches, and the interaction of tumor cells with bone cells, which disturbs normal bone homeostasis and causes the resorbed bone matrix to release signals that encourage the growth of the skeletal tumor. The bone marrow is a remarkably accessible and nourishing nest for DTC, and the bone marrow microenvironment, the cradle of haematopoiesis, is rich in growth factors and cytokines that typically support stem cell activity in the haematopoietic and mesenchymal spectrum (Brizzi, Tarone, and Defilippi 2012; Azevedo et al., 2015). Thus, the bone marrow ecological niche of DTC is similar to that of haematopoietic and mesenchymal stem cells. Cancer cells may exploit these ecological niches' unique homeostatic and regenerative functions to promote their survival and development.

Bone Homeostasis

Bone is a vital organ that plays a complex physiological role, which includes functions such as haematopoiesis and osteogenesis (Florencio-Silva et al., 2015). The intricate skeletal microenvironment is maintained by a dynamic balance between stem cells, progenitor cells, mature immune cells, and supporting stromal cells, called the bone niche (Comazzetto, Shen, and Morrison 2021). The best known are the osteoblasts and osteoclasts involved in bone remodelling, the dynamic balance between which maintains structural integrity and bone health, and the osteocytes that regulate the bone remodelling process in response to mechanical signals and systemic hormones. Osteoblasts and osteoclasts are responsible for the production and resorption of bone, respectively, and bone lining cells account for over 70% of the cells covering the bone surface of the endosteum. Also, bone marrow endothelial cells, adipocytes, and the immune environment regulate bone homeostasis (Croucher, McDonald, and Martin 2016).

The bone matrix, an essential component of the skeleton, is composed of inorganic salts and organic substrates that provide structural support for the associated cells and contain many growth factors that play an essential role in maintaining skeletal homeostasis. Tumor cells in the skeletal environment are capable of causing the formation of skeletal lesions in which new bone is deposited, mainly through the secretion of factors that activate osteoblasts to carry out this biological process. The best known of these is endothelin-1 (ET-1), shown in previous studies to be a significant mediator of osteosclerosis and stimulate osteoblast proliferation (Alam et al., 1992; Chiao et al., 2000; Logothetis and Lin 2005).

Breast and prostate cancer cells can advance osteogenic bone metastases by secreting BMPs, which can be produced by passaged breast and prostate cancer cells (Dai et al., 2008; Dai et al., 2005; Katsuno et al., 2008; Lee et al., 2011). In addition, tumor cells can also express several other osteoblastic regulatory factors, such as FGFs and VEGF, which regulate osteoblastic differentiation (Kitagawa et al., 2005; Li et al., 2008; Siclari et al., 2014). There are also several factors that tumor cells are able to secrete, such as PTHrP, lysophosphatidic acid (LPA), macrophage-stimulating protein (MSP), prostaglandin (PG) E2, IL-8, and granulocyte-macrophage colony-stimulating factor, which further stimulate osteoblast activity and bone resorption (Bendre et al., 2002; Clézardin et al., 2021; Guise et al., 1996; Ouellet et al., 2011; Thomas et al., 1999; Weilbaecher, Guise, and McCauley 2011). When the intrinsic balance of bone physiology is disrupted, these factors can create structural defects and a more favourable environment for metastases caused by different primary tumor types.

Premetastatic Niche

Circulating tumor cells (CTCs) must enter secondary or distant organ locations for metastasis to occur; however, the local microenvironment that CTCs come into contact with during this process has a significant impact on whether or not tumor cell colonization may take place. Before reaching distant organs, primary tumors can be "prepped" for tumor cell colonization in the local microenvironment of those organs. Our understanding of tumor metastasis is aided by the "seed and soil" idea, which also offers a convincing explanation for organ tropism during metastasis: Certain organ areas (the "soil") where the microenvironment is favorable for metastasis are colonized by pro-metastatic tumor cells ("seeds") (Castaño et al., 2018; Catena et al., 2013; Liu and Cao 2016; Peinado et al., 2017).

Previous studies have confirmed that primary tumors can promote metastasis by inducing the formation of a supportive microenvironment at secondary organ sites (known as pre-metastatic niches). The effect of breast cancer on the bone marrow niches begins even before DTC reaches the bone, as xenograft breast tumors secrete lysyl oxidase (LOX), which produces systemic effects and activates osteoclastogenesis, thereby triggering the formation of osteolytic lesions after cancer cell seeding(Cox et al., 2015). The concept of pre-metastatic niches was first introduced by Dr. Lyden and colleagues (Kaplan et al., 2005), who demonstrated that Before the arrival of tumor cells, bone marrow-derived VEGF receptor 1 (VEGFR-1)-positive haematopoietic cells are mobilised by vascular endothelial growth factor (VEGF)-A and placental growth factor (PlGF) secreted by the primary tumor and thus enter the lung (Figure 1). It has been reported that exosomes from primary tumors can act directly on metastatic sites and thus promote subsequent colonisation in an organ-specific manner(Hoshino et al., 2015).

Previous findings suggest that the molecular mechanisms involved in the formation of pre-metastatic niches in the bone can be divided into two categories, some of which are already present in normal bone marrow (Ottewell 2016; Ottewell, Wang, Brown, et al., 2014; Ottewell, Wang, Meek, et al., 2014), while the other requires stimulation by systemic signals from the primary tumor to initiate them (Taverna et al., 2017; Tulotta et al., 2019; Xu et al., 2018). For example, senescent osteoblasts are able to promote the formation of osteoclast differentiation through secreted interleukin (IL)-6, and osteoclast-mediated hyper-resorption of bone, in turn, increases the formation of bone metastases from tumor cells. In addition, the primary tumor secretes factors, such as IL-1b, that can target the stroma and osteoblasts for their future metastatic colonisation of the bone marrow (Tulotta et al., 2019).

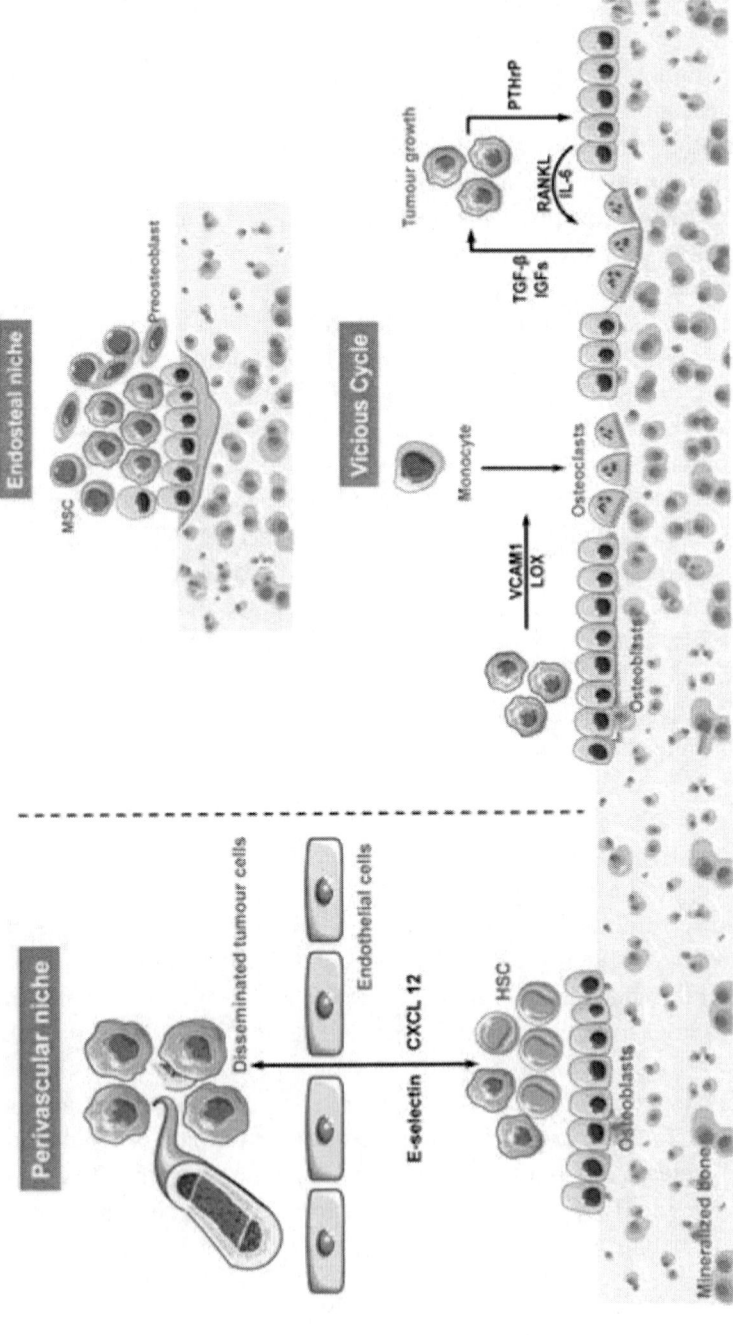

Figure 1. The bone microenvironment and disseminated tumor cells metastasis progression.

In conclusion, previous studies have amply demonstrated that primary tumors already affect and modify the bone marrow niches before metastasis occurs, and further studies on their functional impact on subsequent metastatic seeding and colonisation are needed to develop drugs that target the pre-metastatic niches and provide early treatment options for patients with bone metastases.

The Perivascular Niche

The vascular endothelium that makes up the blood arteries (known as sinusoids) in the bone marrow is fenestrated, which makes it easier for hemopoietic stem cells to be transported (HSCs) (Price et al., 2016). Previous studies have shown that tumor cells hijack the molecular mechanisms of haematopoietic stem cells. Endothelial cell selectin (E-selectin) and CXCL-12 expression on sinusoidal endothelial cells play key roles in homing HSCs in the bone marrow (Sipkins et al., 2005). Bone marrow endothelial cells expressing E-selectin and CXCL-12 have been shown to control how breast and prostate cancer cells adhere by interacting with E-selectin ligands and CXCR-4, respectively (Reymond, d'Água, and Ridley 2013). In addition, the interaction between thrombospondin-1 (TSP1) and TGF-β/periostin decisively regulates the fate of tumor cell quiescence and proliferation. Notably, the interaction of cancer cells with the perivascular niche also makes them chemoresistant (Carlson et al., 2019).

It's interesting to note that despite the tremendous degree of vascularization in bone, the absolute oxygen tension in the bone marrow is not very high. This is most pronounced in the perivascular area, where hypoxia encourages the spread of metastatic disease. Previous studies have demonstrated that HIF-1a plays a regulatory role in bone metastasis and that HIF-1a not only promotes the degree of bone destruction and vascularisation of bone metastases but also directly regulates the expression of the transcription factor TWIST in human breast cancer cells, thereby promoting tumor cell invasion and cancer-induced bone destruction (Yang et al., 2008; Hiraga et al., 2007). A more precise distribution of DTC and HSC and the molecular composition of the corresponding ecological niches could further advance the study of perivascular ecological niches and thus provide a theoretical basis for clinical treatment.

The Endosteal Niche

The endosteal niche is located near the endosteum or the inner layer of the bone marrow cavity in the adult skeleton. It primarily consists of osteoblasts that have not undergone differentiation, such as spindle-shaped N-cadherin1/CD45 osteoblast (SNO) cells (Brizzi, Tarone, and Defilippi 2012; Parfitt et al., 1996; Haug et al., 2008). While tumor cells have the ability to take over the molecular processes used by haematopoietic stem cells, endosteal niches play a crucial role in tolerating and maintaining HSC. Via particular N-cadherin/E-cadherin contacts and connexin-43 (Cx43) gap junctions, SNO cells help ER-positive breast cancer cells survive in a mouse model where tumor cells are injected intra-arterially into the bone. In this microenvironment, DTCs can promote micrometastasis progression by activating mammalian targets of rapamycin (mTOR) signaling and calcium signaling pathways (Wang et al., 2018).

It's interesting to note that in these various bone metastatic tumors, the relative importance of these niches/molecules to tumor cell dormancy differs slightly. It has been shown that endosteal niches provide an environment that supports the survival and growth of breast cancer cells while enabling tumor cells to acquire genetic alterations (e.g., PIK3CA mutations) (Wang et al., 2018; Werner-Klein et al., 2020). In prostate cancer, the interaction between CXCR-4/CXCL-12 and Annexin 2 (ANXA2)/CXCL12 plays a crucial role in the recruitment of tumor cells to the endosteal niche.

In contrast, a dynamic equilibrium between the expression levels of TYRO3 and AXL/MER controls the dormancy of prostate cancer cells in the bone marrow (Khoo et al., 2019). Therefore, more clinical samples need to be used to confirm the mechanism of action of niches and chemicals on the dormancy of tumor cells in various bone metastasis malignancies. There is some intersection between perivascular niches and endosteal niches, meaning that perivascular niches have the potential to be converted into osteogenic niches (Crisan et al., 2008). Bone metabolism may alter the dynamics of both niches and enhance their crosstalk, meaning that DTCs have the potential to alter the cell fate of their neighbors (Muscarella et al., 2021).

The Vicious Cycle

The concept of "vicious circle" was first introduced by Dr. Gregory Mundy and others and referred to as the feed-forward loop between osteoblasts and osteoclasts in advanced pathogenic bone metastases (Mundy 1997). This vicious circle has four main features:

1) Osteoblasts in the bone lining respond to signals from metastases and are regulated to promote proliferation and differentiation further. These signals include parathyroid hormone-related protein (PTHrP), Wnt, bone morphogenetic protein (BMP), fibroblast growth factors such as FGF-9, endothelin, interleukin (IL), and epidermal growth factor receptor (EGFR) ligands, which are associated with the development of osteolytic and osteogenic lesions (Yin et al., 2003; Dai et al., 2008; Bendre et al., 2005; Bendre et al., 2003).
2) Osteoblasts in the bone lining express osteoclastogenic factors in response to signals from the metastases (Guise 1997).
3) In the presence of RANKL, these precursors mature into multinucleated osteoclasts with bone resorption functions.
4) The bone matrix is rich in several growth factors, such as transforming growth factor β (TGFβ) and insulin-like growth factor-I (IGF-I), which are released to participate in this vicious cycle as the osteoclasts become hyper-competent in bone resorption (Lynch 2011).

These findings provide new therapeutic targets for treating patients with advanced bone metastases.

Conclusion

Bone is one of the most common sites of metastasis, with bone metastases most commonly seen in breast, prostate, and lung cancers. Patients with advanced cancer are drastically impacted by these bone metastases. Hence, it is crucial to look into the pathophysiology of bone metastases and use this information as a foundation for creating therapeutic interventions in order to enhance the treatment and prevention of bone metastases and to determine the likelihood that the disease will return. Tumor bone metastases are a succession of progressive events that occur: 1) the formation of pre-metastatic niches capable of attracting circulating tumor cells, 2) the extravasation of attracted tumor cells and their homing to the pre-metastatic niche, and 3) the gradual transformation of the pre-metastatic niche into a metastatic niche that favours the survival of these tumor cells when they have completed their colonisation (Clézardin et al., 2021).

In this chapter, we discussed the biological process of tumor bone metastasis from the pre-metastatic niche to the malignant cycle after DTCs have reached the bone and bone marrow, in which the interaction of different ecological niches with DTCs provides ideas for the different stages of treatment. These findings have already provided therapeutic tools like bisphosphonates and the RANK ligand inhibitor denosumab. The key questions at this stage are what factors lead to the induction of tumor cell dormancy and the interactions of those that activate tumor cell proliferation and metastatic growth. Furthermore, the question remains about which factors or conditions alter the signalling interactions over time to allow dormant cells to awaken.

More studies in this area are believed to provide a good solution for the early diagnosis and treatment of tumor metastases. Future research needs to define more precisely the impact of different niches on the biological process of tumor bone metastasis in the context of clinical cases, which could lead to new mechanistic insights and therapeutic targets. Another promising avenue of research is the treatment of existing skeletal lesions by restoring the metabolic function of osteoblasts. Finally, studies targeting bone markers have the potential to provide critical information for predicting the risk of disease recurrence in cancer patients.

References

Alam, A. S., A. Gallagher, V. Shankar, M. A. Ghatei, H. K. Datta, C. L. Huang, B. S. Moonga, T. J. Chambers, S. R. Bloom, and M. Zaidi. 1992. 'Endothelin inhibits osteoclastic bone resorption by a direct effect on cell motility: implications for the vascular control of bone resorption', *Endocrinology*, 130: 3617-24.

Azevedo, A. S., G. Follain, S. Patthabhiraman, S. Harlepp, and J. G. Goetz. 2015. 'Metastasis of circulating tumor cells: favorable soil or suitable biomechanics, or both?', *Cell Adh. Migr.*, 9: 345-56.

Bendre, M. S., A. G. Margulies, B. Walser, N. S. Akel, S. Bhattacharrya, R. A. Skinner, F. Swain, V. Ramani, K. S. Mohammad, L. L. Wessner, A. Martinez, T. A. Guise, J. M. Chirgwin, D. Gaddy, and L. J. Suva. 2005. 'Tumor-derived interleukin-8 stimulates osteolysis independent of the receptor activator of nuclear factor-kappaB ligand pathway,' *Cancer Res*, 65: 11001-9.

Bendre, M. S., D. Gaddy-Kurten, T. Mon-Foote, N. S. Akel, R. A. Skinner, R. W. Nicholas, and L. J. Suva. 2002. 'Expression of interleukin 8 and not parathyroid hormone-related protein by human breast cancer cells correlates with bone metastasis *in vivo*', *Cancer Res.*, 62: 5571-9.

Bendre, M., D. Gaddy, R. W. Nicholas, and L. J. Suva. 2003. 'Breast cancer metastasis to bone: it is not all about PTHrP', *Clin. Orthop. Relat. Res.*: S39-45.

Brizzi, M. F., G. Tarone, and P. Defilippi. 2012. 'Extracellular matrix, integrins, and growth factors as tailors of the stem cell niche', *Curr. Opin. Cell Biol.*, 24: 645-51.

Carlson, P., A. Dasgupta, C. A. Grzelak, J. Kim, A. Barrett, I. M. Coleman, R. E. Shor, E. T. Goddard, J. Dai, E. M. Schweitzer, A. R. Lim, S. B. Crist, D. A. Cheresh, P. S. Nelson, K. C. Hansen, and C. M. Ghajar. 2019. 'Targeting the perivascular niche sensitizes disseminated tumor cells to chemotherapy,' *Nat. Cell Biol.*, 21: 238-50.

Castaño, Z., B. P. San Juan, A. Spiegel, A. Pant, M. J. DeCristo, T. Laszewski, J. M. Ubellacker, S. R. Janssen, A. Dongre, F. Reinhardt, A. Henderson, A. G. Del Rio, A. M. Gifford, Z. T. Herbert, J. N. Hutchinson, R. A. Weinberg, C. L. Chaffer, and S. S. McAllister. 2018. 'IL-1β inflammatory response driven by primary breast cancer prevents metastasis-initiating cell colonization', *Nat. Cell Biol.*, 20: 1084-97.

Catena, R., N. Bhattacharya, T. El Rayes, S. Wang, H. Choi, D. Gao, S. Ryu, N. Joshi, D. Bielenberg, S. B. Lee, S. A. Haukaas, K. Gravdal, O. J. Halvorsen, L. A. Akslen, R. S. Watnick, and V. Mittal. 2013. 'Bone marrow-derived Gr1+ cells can generate a metastasis-resistant microenvironment via induced secretion of thrombospondin-1', *Cancer Discov.*, 3: 578-89.

Chaffer, C. L., B. P. San Juan, E. Lim, and R. A. Weinberg. 2016. 'EMT, cell plasticity and metastasis', *Cancer Metastasis Rev.*, 35: 645-54.

Chiao, J. W., B. S. Moonga, Y. M. Yang, R. Kancherla, A. Mittelman, J. R. Wu-Wong, and T. Ahmed. 2000. 'Endothelin-1 from prostate cancer cells is enhanced by bone contact which blocks osteoclastic bone resorption', *Br. J. Cancer*, 83: 360-5.

Clarke, B. 2008. 'Normal bone anatomy and physiology', *Clin. J. Am. Soc. Nephrol.*, 3 Suppl 3: S131-9.

Clézardin, P., R. Coleman, M. Puppo, P. Ottewell, E. Bonnelye, F. Paycha, C. B. Confavreux, and I. Holen. 2021. 'Bone metastasis: mechanisms, therapies, and biomarkers', *Physiol. Rev.*, 101: 797-855.

Comazzetto, S., B. Shen, and S. J. Morrison. 2021. 'Niches that regulate stem cells and hematopoiesis in adult bone marrow', *Dev. Cell*, 56: 1848-60.

Cox, T. R., R. M. H. Rumney, E. M. Schoof, L. Perryman, A. M. Høye, A. Agrawal, D. Bird, N. A. Latif, H. Forrest, H. R. Evans, I. D. Huggins, G. Lang, R. Linding, A. Gartland, and J. T. Erler. 2015. 'The hypoxic cancer secretome induces pre-metastatic bone lesions through lysyl oxidase,' *Nature*, 522: 106-10.

Crisan, M., S. Yap, L. Casteilla, C. W. Chen, M. Corselli, T. S. Park, G. Andriolo, B. Sun, B. Zheng, L. Zhang, C. Norotte, P. N. Teng, J. Traas, R. Schugar, B. M. Deasy, S. Badylak, H. J. Buhring, J. P. Giacobino, L. Lazzari, J. Huard, and B. Péault. 2008. 'A perivascular origin for mesenchymal stem cells in multiple human organs', *Cell Stem Cell*, 3: 301-13.

Croucher, P. I., M. M. McDonald, and T. J. Martin. 2016. 'Bone metastasis: the importance of the neighbourhood', *Nat. Rev. Cancer*, 16: 373-86.

Dai, J., C. L. Hall, J. Escara-Wilke, A. Mizokami, J. M. Keller, and E. T. Keller. 2008. 'Prostate cancer induces bone metastasis through Wnt-induced bone morphogenetic protein-dependent and independent mechanisms', *Cancer Res.*, 68: 5785-94.

Dai, J., J. Keller, J. Zhang, Y. Lu, Z. Yao, and E. T. Keller. 2005. 'Bone morphogenetic protein-6 promotes osteoblastic prostate cancer bone metastases through a dual mechanism', *Cancer Res.*, 65: 8274-85.

Florencio-Silva, R., G. R. Sasso, E. Sasso-Cerri, M. J. Simões, and P. S. Cerri. 2015. 'Biology of Bone Tissue: Structure, Function, and Factors That Influence Bone Cells,' *Biomed Res. Int.*, 2015: 421746.

Guise, T. A. 1997. 'Parathyroid hormone-related protein and bone metastases,' *Cancer*, 80: 1572-80.

Guise, T. A., J. J. Yin, S. D. Taylor, Y. Kumagai, M. Dallas, B. F. Boyce, T. Yoneda, and G. R. Mundy. 1996. 'Evidence for a causal role of parathyroid hormone-related protein in the pathogenesis of human breast cancer-mediated osteolysis,' *J. Clin. Invest.*, 98: 1544-9.

Gupta, G. P., and J. Massagué. 2006. 'Cancer metastasis: building a framework,' *Cell*, 127: 679-95.

Haug, J. S., X. C. He, J. C. Grindley, J. P. Wunderlich, K. Gaudenz, J. T. Ross, A. Paulson, K. P. Wagner, Y. Xie, R. Zhu, T. Yin, J. M. Perry, M. J. Hembree, E. P. Redenbaugh, G. L. Radice, C. Seidel, and L. Li. 2008. 'N-cadherin expression level distinguishes reserved versus primed states of hematopoietic stem cells', *Cell Stem Cell*, 2: 367-79.

Hiraga, T., S. Kizaka-Kondoh, K. Hirota, M. Hiraoka, and T. Yoneda. 2007. 'Hypoxia and hypoxia-inducible factor-1 expression enhance osteolytic bone metastases of breast cancer', *Cancer Res*, 67: 4157-63.

Hoshino, A., B. Costa-Silva, T. L. Shen, G. Rodrigues, A. Hashimoto, M. Tesic Mark, et al. 2015. 'Tumor exosome integrins determine organotropic metastasis,' *Nature*, 527: 329-35.

Kang, Y., and K. Pantel. 2013. 'Tumor cell dissemination: emerging biological insights from animal models and cancer patients', *Cancer Cell*, 23: 573-81.

Kaplan, R. N., R. D. Riba, S. Zacharoulis, A. H. Bramley, L. Vincent, C. Costa, et al. 2005. 'VEGFR1-positive haematopoietic bone marrow progenitors initiate the pre-metastatic niche,' *Nature*, 438: 820-7.

Katsuno, Y., A. Hanyu, H. Kanda, Y. Ishikawa, F. Akiyama, T. Iwase, E. Ogata, S. Ehata, K. Miyazono, and T. Imamura. 2008. 'Bone morphogenetic protein signaling enhances invasion and bone metastasis of breast cancer cells through Smad pathway,' *Oncogene*, 27: 6322-33.

Khoo, W. H., G. Ledergor, A. Weiner, D. L. Roden, R. L. Terry, M. M. McDonald, et al. 2019. 'A niche-dependent myeloid transcriptome signature defines dormant myeloma cells.' *Blood*, 134: 30-43.

Kim, J. M., C. Lin, Z. Stavre, M. B. Greenblatt, and J. H. Shim. 2020. 'Osteoblast-Osteoclast Communication and Bone Homeostasis', *Cells*, 9.

Kingsley, L. A., P. G. Fournier, J. M. Chirgwin, and T. A. Guise. 2007. 'Molecular biology of bone metastasis', *Mol. Cancer Ther.*, 6: 2609-17.

Kitagawa, Y., J. Dai, J. Zhang, J. M. Keller, J. Nor, Z. Yao, and E. T. Keller. 2005. 'Vascular endothelial growth factor contributes to prostate cancer-mediated osteoblastic activity', *Cancer Res.*, 65: 10921-9.

Lee, Y. C., C. J. Cheng, M. A. Bilen, J. F. Lu, R. L. Satcher, L. Y. Yu-Lee, G. E. Gallick, S. N. Maity, and S. H. Lin. 2011. 'BMP4 promotes prostate tumor growth in bone through osteogenesis', *Cancer Res.*, 71: 5194-203.

Li, Z. G., P. Mathew, J. Yang, M. W. Starbuck, A. J. Zurita, J. Liu, et al. 2008. 'Androgen receptor-negative human prostate cancer cells induce osteogenesis in mice through FGF9-mediated mechanisms,' *J. Clin. Invest.*, 118: 2697-710.

Liu, Y., and X. Cao. 2016. 'Characteristics and Significance of the Pre-metastatic Niche,' *Cancer Cell*, 30: 668-81.

Logothetis, C. J., and S. H. Lin. 2005. 'Osteoblasts in prostate cancer metastasis to bone', *Nat Rev. Cancer*, 5: 21-8.

Lynch, C. C. 2011. 'Matrix metalloproteinases as master regulators of the vicious cycle of bone metastasis', *Bone*, 48: 44-53.

Mundy, G. R. 1997. 'Mechanisms of bone metastasis', *Cancer*, 80: 1546-56.

Mundy, G. R. 2002. 'Metastasis to bone: causes, consequences and therapeutic opportunities', *Nat. Rev. Cancer*, 2: 584-93.

Muscarella, A. M., S. Aguirre, X. Hao, S. M. Waldvogel, and X. H. Zhang. 2021. 'Exploiting bone niches: progression of disseminated tumor cells to metastasis,' *J. Clin. Invest.*, 131.

Ottewell, P. D. 2016. 'The role of osteoblasts in bone metastasis', *J. Bone Oncol.*, 5: 124-27.

Ottewell, P. D., N. Wang, H. K. Brown, K. J. Reeves, C. A. Fowles, P. I. Croucher, C. L. Eaton, and I. Holen. 2014. 'Zoledronic acid has differential antitumor activity in the pre- and postmenopausal bone microenvironment *in vivo*', *Clin. Cancer Res.*, 20: 2922-32.

Ottewell, P. D., N. Wang, J. Meek, C. A. Fowles, P. I. Croucher, C. L. Eaton, and I. Holen. 2014. 'Castration-induced bone loss triggers growth of disseminated prostate cancer cells in bone', *Endocr. Relat. Cancer*, 21: 769-81.

Ouellet, V., K. Tiedemann, A. Mourskaia, J. E. Fong, D. Tran-Thanh, E. Amir, M. Clemons, B. Perbal, S. V. Komarova, and P. M. Siegel. 2011. 'CCN3 impairs osteoblast and stimulates osteoclast differentiation to favor breast cancer metastasis to bone', *Am. J. Pathol.*, 178: 2377-88.

Pantel, K., R. H. Brakenhoff, and B. Brandt. 2008. 'Detection, clinical relevance and specific biological properties of disseminating tumor cells', *Nat. Rev. Cancer*, 8: 329-40.

Parfitt, A. M., G. R. Mundy, G. D. Roodman, D. E. Hughes, and B. F. Boyce. 1996. 'A new model for the regulation of bone resorption, with particular reference to the effects of bisphosphonates', *J. Bone Miner. Res.*, 11: 150-9.

Peinado, H., H. Zhang, I. R. Matei, B. Costa-Silva, A. Hoshino, G. Rodrigues, B. Psaila, R. N. Kaplan, J. F. Bromberg, Y. Kang, M. J. Bissell, T. R. Cox, A. J. Giaccia, J. T. Erler, S. Hiratsuka, C. M. Ghajar, and D. Lyden. 2017. 'Pre-metastatic niches: organ-specific homes for metastases,' *Nat. Rev. Cancer*, 17: 302-17.

Price, T. T., M. L. Burness, A. Sivan, M. J. Warner, R. Cheng, C. H. Lee, L. Olivere, K. Comatas, J. Magnani, H. Kim Lyerly, Q. Cheng, C. M. McCall, and D. A. Sipkins. 2016. 'Dormant breast cancer micrometastases reside in specific bone marrow niches that regulate their transit to and from bone,' *Sci. Transl. Med.*, 8: 340ra73.

Puisieux, A., T. Brabletz, and J. Caramel. 2014. 'Oncogenic roles of EMT-inducing transcription factors', *Nat. Cell Biol.*, 16: 488-94.

Reymond, N., B. B. d'Água, and A. J. Ridley. 2013. 'Crossing the endothelial barrier during metastasis', *Nat. Rev. Cancer*, 13: 858-70.

Rodan, G. A. 1998. 'Bone homeostasis', *Proc. Natl. Acad. Sc.i U S A*, 95: 13361-2.

Siclari, V. A., K. S. Mohammad, D. R. Tompkins, H. Davis, C. R. McKenna, X. Peng, L. L. Wessner, M. Niewolna, T. A. Guise, A. Suvannasankha, and J. M. Chirgwin. 2014. 'Tumor-expressed adrenomedullin accelerates breast cancer bone metastasis', *Breast Cancer Res.*, 16: 458.

Sipkins, D. A., X. Wei, J. W. Wu, J. M. Runnels, D. Côté, T. K. Means, A. D. Luster, D. T. Scadden, and C. P. Lin. 2005. 'In vivo imaging of specialized bone marrow endothelial microdomains for tumor engraftment', *Nature*, 435: 969-73.

Taverna, S., M. Pucci, M. Giallombardo, M. A. Di Bella, M. Santarpia, P. Reclusa, I. Gil-Bazo, C. Rolfo, and R. Alessandro. 2017. 'Amphiregulin contained in NSCLC-exosomes induces osteoclast differentiation through the activation of EGFR pathway,' *Sci. Rep.*, 7: 3170.

Thomas, R. J., T. A. Guise, J. J. Yin, J. Elliott, N. J. Horwood, T. J. Martin, and M. T. Gillespie. 1999. 'Breast cancer cells interact with osteoblasts to support osteoclast formation', *Endocrinology*, 140: 4451-8.

Tulotta, C., D. V. Lefley, K. Freeman, W. M. Gregory, A. M. Hanby, P. R. Heath, et al. 2019. 'Endogenous Production of IL1B by Breast Cancer Cells Drives Metastasis and Colonization of the Bone Microenvironment', *Clin. Cancer Res.*, 25: 2769-82.

Wang, H., L. Tian, J. Liu, A. Goldstein, I. Bado, W. Zhang, B. R. Arenkiel, Z. Li, M. Yang, S. Du, H. Zhao, D. R. Rowley, S. T. C. Wong, Z. Gugala, and X. H. Zhang. 2018. 'The Osteogenic Niche Is a Calcium Reservoir of Bone Micrometastases and Confers Unexpected Therapeutic Vulnerability', *Cancer Cell*, 34: 823-39.e7.

Weilbaecher, K. N., T. A. Guise, and L. K. McCauley. 2011. 'Cancer to bone: a fatal attraction', *Nat. Rev. Cancer*, 11: 411-25.

Werner-Klein, M., A. Grujovic, C. Irlbeck, M. Obradović, M. Hoffmann, H. Koerkel-Qu, et al. 2020. 'Interleukin-6 trans-signaling is a candidate mechanism to drive progression of human DCCs during clinical latency', *Nat. Commun.*, 11: 4977.

Xu, Z., X. Liu, H. Wang, J. Li, L. Dai, J. Li, and C. Dong. 2018. 'Lung adenocarcinoma cell-derived exosomal miR-21 facilitates osteoclastogenesis', *Gene*, 666: 116-22.

Yang, M. H., M. Z. Wu, S. H. Chiou, P. M. Chen, S. Y. Chang, C. J. Liu, S. C. Teng, and K. J. Wu. 2008. 'Direct regulation of TWIST by HIF-1alpha promotes metastasis', *Nat. Cell Biol.*, 10: 295-305.

Yin, J. J., K. S. Mohammad, S. M. Käkönen, S. Harris, J. R. Wu-Wong, J. L. Wessale, R. J. Padley, I. R. Garrett, J. M. Chirgwin, and T. A. Guise. 2003. 'A causal role for endothelin-1 in the pathogenesis of osteoblastic bone metastases', *Proc. Natl. Acad. Sci. U S A*, 100: 10954-9.

Chapter 6

Macrophages' Promotion of Bone Metastasis

Zhiguo Ling[1]
and Yueqi Chen[2,*]

[1] Institute of Immunology,
Third Military Medical University (Army Medical University),
Chongqing, People's Republic of China
[2] Department of Orthopedics, Southwest Hospital,
Third Military Medical University (Army Medical University),
Chongqing, People's Republic of China

Abstract

Bone metastasis is a major cause of cancer-related mortality and treatment failure. Current strategies for treating bone metastasis are primarily aimed at relieving symptoms and slowing the progression of the disease, which fails to produce effective therapeutic outcomes. Therefore, it is critical to develop highly effective and promising therapeutic strategies.

Macrophages are the primary component of the tumor micro-environment and are key to tumor growth, invasion, and distant metastasis. Disruption of bone homeostasis is often a result of bone metastasis and thus restoring bone homeostasis is essential for successful treatment. Targeting macrophages may be a potential therapeutic option for restoring bone homeostasis due to their role as regulators. In addition, compelling clinical and scientific evidence has shown that macrophages could facilitate the multi-step progression of bone metastasis. Intriguingly, macrophages interact not only with cancer cells but also with local stromal cells, such as osteoclasts and osteoblasts, within the

---

* Corresponding Author's Email: chenyueqi1012@sina.com.

In: New Research on Bone Metastasis
Editor: Joseph Gerfried
ISBN: 979-8-88697-799-8
© 2023 Nova Science Publishers, Inc.

bone microenvironment, resulting in further bone metastasis deterioration.

In this chapter, we provide an overview of the pivotal role macrophages play in bone metastasis, as well as discuss promising strategies for targeting macrophages for bone metastasis treatment.

Keywords: macrophages, bone metastasis, bone homeostasis, TAMs, immunotherapy

Introduction

Bone is a common site of metastasis for numerous cancer types, especially those of the lung cancer, breast cancer, and prostate cancer [1]. Skeletal-related events caused by bone metastasis, such as pathological fractures and cancer-induced bone pain, result in increased mortality, reduced quality of life for patients, and increased medical as well as economic burdens for society. However, current clinical therapies for bone metastasis, such as endocrine therapy, chemoradiotherapy, and open surgery, are only aimed at palliating symptoms and arresting disease progression, thus making it difficult to satisfy medical needs [2]. With the emergence of an ever-growing number of immunotherapy targets, immunological cancer therapy appears to be a superior option for the current treatment of tumor metastasis [3]. Consequently, the exploration of novel immunotherapeutic targets is essential for the study of bone metastasis treatment.

Macrophages are a pivotal component of intrinsic immunity, tasked with engulfing cellular debris, defending against exogenous pathogens, and initiating specific immune responses. However, due to their plasticity, macrophages may not always act as a 'policeman.' In response to various environmental stimuli, macrophages undergo distinct polarization pathways, giving rise to diverse subpopulations with distinct phenotypes and functional characteristics [4]. Generally, the phenotypes of macrophages are classified into M1 and M2, with the latter further subdivided into M2a, M2b, M2c, and M2d.

Macrophages infiltrating the tumor tissue are referred to as tumor associated macrophages (TAMs), and compelling evidence suggests that TAMs are the most abundant immune cells in the tumor microenvironment, accounting for around 50% of the tumor mass. Moreover, TAMs play a pivotal role in the process of tumor invasion and metastasis [5]. Additionally, macrophages could regulate bone homeostasis, which may be linked to metastatic tumor growth in the bone microenvironment [6]. Therefore, recent research on the regulation of macrophages in bone metastasis has prompted exploration into novel immunotherapies for bone metastasis. Collectively, macrophages may contribute to bone metastasis, thus making future research into novel therapies for bone metastasis of paramount importance, with the relationship between macrophages and bone metastasis potentially yielding new breakthroughs.

Herein, we review the mechanisms involved in the regulation of bone homeostasis by macrophages, the role of macrophages in the growth as well as metastasis of breast cancer and prostate cancer, and how macrophages contribute to bone metastasis cascade. In addition, we will provide an outlook on targeted macrophages therapy strategies for the treatment of bone metastasis and discuss potential clinical applications.

Macrophages' Actions on Bone Homeostasis

Traditionally, macrophages were only derived from circulating monocytes, however, recent evidence has suggested that tissue-resident macrophages originate from yolk-sac-derived erythro-myeloid progenitors [7]. However, tissue-resident macrophages could not only be established prior to birth and remain throughout adulthood via longevity and self-renewal, but they could also be supplemented by adult monocyte-derived macrophages. Due to their plasticity, tissue-resident macrophages exhibit significant phenotypic variability in different tissues, which is reflected in their function as well as morphology [4]. Under physiological conditions, most macrophages maintain the M0 phenotype to sustain tissue homeostasis, with bones being no exception.

Bone homeostasis is a dynamic balance maintained through bone formation and bone resorption, which is precisely regulated by osteoblasts, osteoclasts, osteocytes, hormones, and cytokines [1]. Osteoblasts are critical contributors to bone formation, responsible for the production, secretion, and mineralization of the bone matrix. Osteoclasts, on the other hand, are tasked with bone resorption. Imbalances in bone homeostasis caused by bone-related diseases, such as bone metastasis, necessitate a re-establishment of equilibrium for effective clinical treatment of said conditions [8]. Interestingly, there are convincing evidence that macrophages are capable of maintaining bone homeostasis, with the crosstalk among osteoblasts, osteoclasts, and macrophages acting as the main regulatory mechanism (Table 1).

Table 1. Functions and relevant mechanisms of macrophages in bone homeostasis

Bone Homeostasis	Functions	Mechanisms	Associated cytokines	References
Bone Resorption	Positive	M1 macrophages decreased OPG expression in BMSCs	N/A	[10]
		M1 macrophages induce osteoclasts differentiation	TNF-α, IL-1β, and IL-6	[11]
		M2 macrophages convert to M1 macrophages for enhancing the function of osteoclasts	TNF-α	[12]
		Macrophages could eliminate by-products of bone resorption during mouse embryonic development	N/A	[16]
		Osteomacs could differentiate into osteoclasts	RANKL, M-CSF	[21]
		Osteomacs could respond timely to bone erosion and initiate osteoclasts recruitment	N/A	[22]
	Negative	M2 macrophages express IL-10 to induce the reduction of RANKL-induced NFATc1 expression	IL-10, NFATc1	[13-15]
Bone Formation	Positive	Osteomacs could secrete BMP that induce the high expression of osteoblasts differentiation genes in BMSCs	BMP	[23]
		Macrophages could promote BMSCs proliferation and enhance alkaline phosphatase activity of BMSCs	N/A	[25]
		Macrophages also generate osteopontin (OPN), TGF-β, and 1,25 dihydroxy-vitamin D3 to directly promote bone formation	OPN, TGF-β, and 1,25 dihydroxy-vitamin D3	[26]

Bone Homeo-stasis	Func-tions	Mechanisms	Associated cytokines	References
	Negative	Macrophages could also negatively regulate osteoblasts function by secreting inflammatory cytokines or growth factors, such as TNF-α and IL-6	TNF-α, IL-6	[27]

The Role of Macrophages in Bone Resorption

Osteoclasts are the main players responsible for bone resorption, and due to their origin from the mononuclear phagocyte system and their bone-specific function, they are regarded as a population of tissue-resident macrophages [9]. In a broad sense, osteoclasts are traditionally thought to be a step in the differentiation of macrophages in the bone microenvironment, thus their role in bone resorption could be argued to be a part of macrophage function. By excluding osteoclasts from the discussion, we can gain a more general understanding of macrophages involvement in bone metastasis.

As elaborated above, macrophages could polarize into M1 phenotype (pro-inflammatory) and M2 phenotype (anti-inflammatory) under different microenvironments. Different types of macrophages have different roles in bone resorption. Lu et al. found that the co-culture of M1 macrophages with bone mesenchymal stem cells (BMSCs) could result in decreased osteoprotegerin (OPG) expression in BMSCs [10]. The decreased expression of OPG by BMSCs due to the presence of M1 macrophages prevents them from inhibiting osteoclasts activation via the OPG/the receptor activator of NF-κB ligand (RANKL) signaling pathway, thereby resulting in increased osteoclasts activity. But the underlying mechanism is still unknown.

Additionally, M1 macrophages could also secrete tumor necrosis factor-α (TNF-α), IL-1β, and IL-6, which could lead to osteoclasts differentiation [11]. TNF-α, in turn, could convert M2 macrophages to M1 macrophages via macrophage-colony stimulating factor (M-CSF), resulting in an increase in osteoclasts activity in a positive feedback loop [12]. M2 macrophages exert anti-inflammatory effects mainly by secreting IL-10, IL-12, chemokine (CC motif) ligand 18 (CCL-18), and CCL-22 [13]. IL-10 could inhibit osteoclasts activity by blocking the production of pro-osteoclastic cytokines, and studies have shown that it could even prevent osteoclasts formation directly by reducing RANKL-induced NFATc1 expression [14, 15]. Moreover, Tosun et al. found that macrophages could eliminate by-products of bone resorption during mouse embryonic development, thereby inducing osteoclastgenesis [16].

In addition to osteoclasts, bone-resident macrophages also include a newly defined subpopulation of macrophages known as bone osteal macrophages (osteomacs). Osteomacs are a characteristic group of macrophages that are positioned close to the surface of cortical bone in direct contact with the bone surface [17]. The specific markers that distinguish macrophages from osteoclasts are F4/80 (+), CD169 (+), CD68 (+), and CD107b (+), but tartrate-resistant acid phosphatase (TRAP$^-$) is the marker that is specifically used to identify osteomacs [18-20]. Osteomacs could be stimulated by RANKL and M-CSF to differentiate into osteoclasts *in vitro*, but not as effectively as the monocyte-macrophage system [21]. In addition, osteomacs could quickly detect bone erosion and trigger the recruitment of osteoclasts, which ultimately leads to increased bone resorption [22].

In conclusion, macrophages play a diverse role in the regulation of bone resorption due to macrophages plasticity. It is essential to elucidate the underlying mechanisms by which osteomacs, M1 macrophages, and M2 macrophages regulate bone resorption in order to gain insight into the development of osteolytic lesions in bone metastasis.

Macrophages' Contribution to Bone Formation

Macrophages are responsible for the production of cytokines and growth factors that are essential for bone formation. Talati et al. observed that osteomacs could secrete bone morphogenetic protein (BMP) that induces the high expression of osteoblasts differentiation genes in BMSCs. Further validation revealed that the osteoblastic differentiation of BMSCs was inhibited by anti-BMP-2 antibody treatment, resulting in the attenuation of osteogenic effect of osteomacs [23]. In the transwell co-culture assay, it was found that osteomacs facilitated the differentiation of BMSCs into osteoblasts and augmented their osteogenic effects *in vitro*. However, M1 and M2 macrophages have different roles, with M1 macrophages inhibiting osteogenesis and M2 macrophages significantly enhancing it [24]. Besides, conditioned medium from macrophages could promote BMSCs proliferation and enhance alkaline phosphatase activity of BMSCs, indicating the differentiation of BMSCs into osteoblasts [25]. Macrophages also generate osteopontin (OPN), TGF-β, and 1,25 dihydroxy-vitamin D3 to directly promote bone formation [26]. Conversely, macrophages could also negatively regulate osteoblasts function by secreting inflammatory cytokines or growth factors, such as TNF-α and IL-6 [27].

Macrophages also contribute to regulate the activity of osteoblasts, and even directly participate in bone formation. It was found that there was a significant decrease of osteomacs in macrophage Fas-induced apoptosis (Mafia) mouse, and even a complete absence of osteoblasts on the bone surface [19]. It suggests that osteomacs may directly regulate the number and function of osteoblasts. In addition to the direct action on osteoblasts, osteomacs could also control bone formation in synergy with other macrophages and osteoclasts [28].

In conclusion, the regulation of macrophages in bone homeostasis is intricate and multifaceted, and the underlying mechanisms are yet to be fully investigated. Reestablishing bone homeostasis is an essential therapeutic objective in the treatment of bone metastasis and making the therapeutic approach of restoring bone homeostasis by targeting macrophages highly promising. However, the prevailing phase of research concerning the role of macrophages in bone homeostasis is not within the context of bone metastasis, so it is essential to elucidate how macrophages regulate bone homeostasis in the bone metastasis microenvironment.

The Function of Macrophages in Bone Metastatic Cascade

Bone metastasis is a sequential multistep process, each of which abounds with macrophages targets and provides an opportunity for the prevention and treatment of bone metastasis. Initially, few primary tumor cells are released and seeded into the pre-metastatic niche (PMN) through epithelial-mesenchymal transition (EMT) and local invasion into the peripheral blood circulation, allowing tumor cells to escape from the primary site [29]. Subsequently, the tumor cells could adapt to the bone marrow microenvironment and initiate tumor cells colonization [30]. Depending on the response of tumor cells to the bone microenvironment, tumor cells could enter a rapid growth phase or a dormant phase. And the dormant tumor cells could be reactivated to enter the growth phase. Eventually, the metastatic tumor cells would grow without any restriction by the bone microenvironment and even modify bone homeostasis [31]. As understanding of the steps involved in bone metastasis continues to increase, numerous therapeutic targets for bone metastasis have been identified, with macrophages being a particularly promising target.

Macrophages display diverse phenotypes in response to different environmental cues, and hence we hypothesize that there are also specific subpopulations of macrophages in the bone metastasis microenvironment. Ma et al. identified a subpopulation of macrophages, termed bone metastasis-associated macrophages (BoMAMs), that promote bone metastasis [32]. They determined, via tracing macrophage precursors, that the infiltrating macrophages in the metastasis were derived from $Ly6C^+CCR2^+$ inflammatory monocytes. Meanwhile, the research also confirmed that BoMAMs exerted enhanced tumor growth depending on CCL2-CCR2 and IL-4R signaling. Besides, Huang et al. suggested that TAMs could express CCL-5 to elevate local invasion and EMT of prostate cancer cells through β-catenin/STAT3 signaling [33]. Thus, targeting TAMs/CCL-5 could potentially suppress the genesis of prostate cancer bone metastasis from the origin.

Furthermore, macrophages also orchestrate the dormant state of breast cancer cells, with distinct macrophage phenotypes having various effects on tumor dormancy. M1 macrophages could secrete exosomes to disrupt dormancy through NF-κB activation; however, exosomes released by M2 macrophages maintain cancer cell dormancy and reduce their proliferation through gap junctional intercellular communication [34]. Moreover, it was reported that abscisic acid could regulate dormancy of prostate cancer cells in bone microenvironment, and abscisic acid is the inducer of polarization of TAMs toward the M1 phenotype [35].

Finally, metastatic tumor cells could disrupt bone homeostasis during the last stage of bone metastasis. Tumor cells could stimulate excessive bone formation to form osteogenic lesions on the one hand, and excessive bone resorption to form osteolysis lesions on the other hand. It appears that macrophages could also partake in the regulation of osteogenic lesions and osteolysis lesions. Mizutani et al. found that prostate cancer cells overexpress CCL-2 to recruit monocytes, which then differentiate into TAMs and osteoclasts [36]. Besides, it has been found that depletion of $CD169^+$ macrophages could mitigate osteogenic lesions caused by prostate cancer [37]. Furthermore, macrophages could also express migration inhibitory factor to recruit osteoclasts, thus augmenting osteolytic lesions [38]. Collectively, macrophages are never absent from any stages of bone metastasis, thus elucidating their function at critical stages may aid in the more precise targeting of treatments for bone metastasis.

Aside from their direct involvement in bone metastasis processes, macrophages could also regulate bone metastasis through other pathways. It is conventionally appreciated that macrophages exert efferocytosis to maintain immune homeostasis, but TAMs maybe promote tumor metastasis with the help of efferocytosis [39]. Roca et al. found that macrophage-driven efferocytosis could trigger the expression of CXCL5 to stimulate bone metastasis within the bone microenvironment [40]. It is reported that macrophages are 'culprits' of resistance to bone metastasis therapy. Androgen deprivation therapy is frequently used to treat bone metastasis caused by prostate cancer, yet most patients are resistant to the therapy. Li et al. found that macrophages could activate the fibronectin (FN1)-integrin alpha 5 (ITGA5) signaling pathway in prostate cancer cells through the secretion of activin A, ultimately leading to resistance to androgen deprivation therapy [41]. Additionally, macrophages could contribute to tumor angiogenesis, immunosuppression, and the primary tumor growth, which in turn promotes bone metastasis [42].

Conclusion and Future Prospectives

Macrophages are the principal immune cells present in the bone metastasis microenvironment, and thus treatments that focus on targeting them are very promising. Due to the extreme plasticity, the functions of macrophages in bone metastasis are similarly very diverse. Patients with bone metastasis often suffer from imbalances in bone homeostasis, manifesting as either osteolytic or osteogenic lesions. Consequently, restoring bone homeostasis is essential. Compelling evidence have demonstrated that M1 macrophages, M2 macrophages, and osteomacs all could regulate bone homeostasis. Bone metastasis is a multi-stage process that includes tumor cells escape, survival, dormancy, reactivation, and modification of bone. Macrophages are involved in multiple stages of bone metastasis and regulate the development of bone metastasis. While some progress has been made in targeting macrophages for the treatment of bone metastasis, research in this field is still very limited. Therefore, it is necessary to further explore the mechanisms by which macrophages impact bone metastasis and the growth of metastatic tumors in the bone microenvironment, in order to devise novel therapeutic strategies that target macrophages.

With the approval of chimeric antigen receptor (CAR)-T cell therapies one after another worldwide, the development of cancer immunotherapy, represented by CAR-T, has brought hope of a cure for hematological malignancies [43]. Consistently, however, in the field of solid tumor treatment, the extremely promising therapeutic strategy does not seem to evolve well. Fortunately, Klichinsky et al. designed human chimeric antigen receptor macrophage (CAR-M) immunotherapy based on the success of CAR-T cell therapies [44]. The advent of CAR-M will undoubtedly lead to a bright future for the treatment of bone metastasis. Moreover, future research is needed to further elucidate the mechanisms underlying the dominant role of macrophages in bone metastasis and to explore macrophage-targeted therapies for the treatment of bone metastasis.

References

[1] Ling Z, Yang C, Tan J, Dou C, Chen Y. Beyond immunosuppressive effects: dual roles of myeloid-derived suppressor cells in bone-related diseases. *Cell Mol. Life Sci.* 78, 7161-7183 (2021).
[2] Coleman R E, Croucher P I, Padhani A R, Clézardin P, Chow E, Fallon M, Guise T, Colangeli S, Capanna R, Costa L. Bone metastases. *Nat. Rev. Dis. Primers* 6, 83 (2020).
[3] Yu B, Baofa B. A New Era of Immuno Surgery is Coming: A Novel Eclectic Approach for Cancer Treatment with Liquid Knife & Immuno Therapy. (2022).
[4] Varol C, Mildner A, Jung S. Macrophages: development and tissue specialization. *Annu. Rev. Immunol.* 33, 643-675 (2015).
[5] Christofides A, Strauss L, Yeo A, Cao C, Charest A, Boussiotis VA. The complex role of tumor-infiltrating macrophages. *Nat Immunol* 23, 1148-1156 (2022).
[6] Bozec A, Soulat D. Latest perspectives on macrophages in bone homeostasis. *Pflugers Arch.* 469, 517-525 (2017).
[7] Gomez Perdiguero E, Klapproth K, Schulz C, Busch K, Azzoni E, Crozet L, Garner H, Trouillet C, de Bruijn MF, Geissmann F, Rodewald HR. Tissue-resident macrophages originate from yolk-sac-derived erythro-myeloid progenitors. *Nature* 518, 547-551 (2015).
[8] 8. Clézardin P, Coleman R, Puppo M, Ottewell P, Bonnelye E, Paycha F, Confavreux CB, Holen I. Bone metastasis: mechanisms, therapies, and biomarkers. *Physiol Rev* 101, 797-855 (2021).
[9] Kotani M, Kikuta J, Klauschen F, Chino T, Kobayashi Y, Yasuda H, Tamai K, Miyawaki A, Kanagawa O, Tomura M, Ishii M. Systemic circulation and bone recruitment of osteoclast precursors tracked by using fluorescent imaging techniques. *J Immunol* 190, 605-612 (2013).
[10] Lu LY, Loi F, Nathan K, Lin T H, Pajarinen J, Gibon E, Nabeshima A, Cordova L, Jämsen E, Yao Z, Goodman SB. Pro-inflammatory M1 macrophages promote Osteogenesis by mesenchymal stem cells via the COX-2-prostaglandin E2 pathway. *J. Orthop. Res.* 35, 2378-2385 (2017).

[11] Jung Y K, Kang Y M, Han S. Osteoclasts in the Inflammatory Arthritis: Implications for Pathologic Osteolysis. *Immune Netw.* 19, e2 (2019).
[12] Zhao Z, Hou X, Yin X, Li Y, Duan R, Boyce B F, Yao Z. TNF Induction of NF-κB RelB Enhances RANKL-Induced Osteoclastogenesis by Promoting Inflammatory Macrophage Differentiation but also Limits It through Suppression of NFATc1 Expression. *PLoS One* 10, e0135728 (2015).
[13] Hu Y, Huang J, Chen C, Wang Y, Hao Z, Chen T, Wang J, Li J. Strategies of Macrophages to Maintain Bone Homeostasis and Promote Bone Repair: A Narrative Review. *J. Funct. Biomater.* 14, (2022).
[14] Tanaka K, Yamagata K, Kubo S, Nakayamada S, Sakata K, Matsui T, Yamagishi SI, Okada Y, Tanaka Y. Glycolaldehyde-modified advanced glycation end-products inhibit differentiation of human monocytes into osteoclasts via upregulation of IL-10. *Bone* 128, 115034 (2019).
[15] Evans K E, Fox S W. Interleukin-10 inhibits osteoclastogenesis by reducing NFATc1 expression and preventing its translocation to the nucleus. *BMC Cell Biol.* 8, 4 (2007).
[16] Tosun B, Wolff L I, Houben A, Nutt S, Hartmann C. Osteoclasts and Macrophages-Their Role in Bone Marrow Cavity Formation During Mouse Embryonic Development. *J. Bone Miner. Res.* 37, 1761-1774 (2022).
[17] Mohamad S F, Xu L, Ghosh J, Childress P J, Abeysekera I, Himes ER, Wu H, Alvarez M B, Davis K M, Aguilar-Perez A, Hong J M, Bruzzaniti A, Kacena M A, Srour E F. Osteomacs interact with megakaryocytes and osteoblasts to regulate murine hematopoietic stem cell function. *Blood Adv.* 1, 2520-2528 (2017).
[18] Cho S W, Soki F N, Koh A J, Eber M R, Entezami P, Park SI, van Rooijen N, McCauley LK. Osteal macrophages support physiologic skeletal remodeling and anabolic actions of parathyroid hormone in bone. *Proc. Natl. Acad. Sci. U S A* 111, 1545-1550 (2014).
[19] Chang M K, Raggatt L J, Alexander K A, Kuliwaba J S, Fazzalari N L, Schroder K, Maylin E R, Ripoll V M, Hume D A, Pettit A R. Osteal tissue macrophages are intercalated throughout human and mouse bone lining tissues and regulate osteoblast function *in vitro* and *in vivo*. *J. Immuno.l* 181, 1232-1244 (2008).
[20] Batoon L, Millard S M, Wullschleger M E, Preda C, Wu A C, Kaur S, Tseng H W, Hume DA, Levesque JP, Raggatt LJ, Pettit AR. CD169(+) macrophages are critical for osteoblast maintenance and promote intramembranous and endochondral ossification during bone repair. *Biomaterials* 196, 51-66 (2019).
[21] Pettit A R, Chang M K, Hume D A, Raggatt LJ. Osteal macrophages: a new twist on coupling during bone dynamics. *Bone* 43, 976-982 (2008).
[22] Batoon L, Millard S M, Raggatt LJ, Pettit AR. Osteomacs and Bone Regeneration. *Curr. Osteoporos. Rep.* 15, 385-395 (2017).
[23] Talati M, West J, Zaynagetdinov R, Hong C C, Han W, Blackwell T, Robinson L, Blackwell TS, Lane K. BMP pathway regulation of and by macrophages. *PLoS One* 9, e94119 (2014).
[24] Gong L, Zhao Y, Zhang Y, Ruan Z. The Macrophage Polarization Regulates MSC Osteoblast Differentiation *in vitro*. *Ann. Clin. Lab. Sci.* 46, 65-71 (2016).

[25] He X T, Li X, Yin Y, Wu R X, Xu X Y, Chen F M. The effects of conditioned media generated by polarized macrophages on the cellular behaviours of bone marrow mesenchymal stem cells. *J. Cell Mol. Med.* 22, 1302-1315 (2018).

[26] Miron R J, Bosshardt D D. OsteoMacs: Key players around bone biomaterials. *Biomaterials* 82, 1-19 (2016).

[27] Harmer D, Falank C, Reagan M R. Interleukin-6 Interweaves the Bone Marrow Microenvironment, Bone Loss, and Multiple Myeloma. *Front. Endocrinol. (Lausanne)* 9, 788 (2018).

[28] Guihard P, Danger Y, Brounais B, David E, Brion R, Delecrin J, Richards C D, Chevalier S, Rédini F, Heymann D, Gascan H, Blanchard F. Induction of osteogenesis in mesenchymal stem cells by activated monocytes/macrophages depends on oncostatin M signaling. *Stem Cells* 30, 762-772 (2012).

[29] Peinado H, Zhang H, Matei I R, Costa-Silva B, Hoshino A, Rodrigues G, Psaila B, Kaplan R N, Bromberg J F, Kang Y, Bissell M J, Cox T R, Giaccia A J, Erler J T, Hiratsuka S, Ghajar C M, Lyden D. Pre-metastatic niches: organ-specific homes for metastases. *Nat. Rev. Cancer* 17, 302-317 (2017).

[30] Liu Y, Cao X. Characteristics and Significance of the Pre-metastatic Niche. *Cancer Cell* 30, 668-681 (2016).

[31] Croucher P I, McDonald M M, Martin T J. Bone metastasis: the importance of the neighbourhood. *Nat. Rev. Cancer* 16, 373-386 (2016).

[32] Ma R Y, Zhang H, Li X F, Zhang C B, Selli C, Tagliavini G, Lam A D, Prost S, Sims AH, Hu HY, Ying T, Wang Z, Ye Z, Pollard JW, Qian BZ. Monocyte-derived macrophages promote breast cancer bone metastasis outgrowth. *J. Exp. Med.* 217, (2020).

[33] Huang R, Wang S, Wang N, Zheng Y, Zhou J, Yang B, Wang X, Zhang J, Guo L, Wang S, Chen Z, Wang Z, Xiang S. CCL5 derived from tumor-associated macrophages promotes prostate cancer stem cells and metastasis via activating β-catenin/STAT3 signaling. *Cell Death Dis.* 11, 234 (2020).

[34] Walker N D, Elias M, Guiro K, Bhatia R, Greco SJ, Bryan M, Gergues M, Sandiford O A, Ponzio N M, Leibovich S J, Rameshwar P. Exosomes from differentially activated macrophages influence dormancy or resurgence of breast cancer cells within bone marrow stroma. *Cell Death Dis.* 10, 59 (2019).

[35] Jeong H, Kim S, Hong B J, Lee C J, Kim Y E, Bok S, Oh J M, Gwak S H, Yoo M Y, Lee M S, Chung S J, Defrêne J, Tessier P, Pelletier M, Jeon H, Roh TY, Kim B, Kim K H, Ju J H, Kim S, Lee Y J, Kim D W, Kim I H, Kim H J, Park J W, Lee Y S, Lee J S, Cheon G J, Weissman I L, Chung D H, Jeon Y K, Ahn G O. Tumor-Associated Macrophages Enhance Tumor Hypoxia and Aerobic Glycolysis. *Cancer Res.* 79, 795-806 (2019).

[36] Mizutani K, Sud S, McGregor N A, Martinovski G, Rice B T, Craig M J, Varsos Z S, Roca H, Pienta K J. The chemokine CCL2 increases prostate tumor growth and bone metastasis through macrophage and osteoclast recruitment. *Neoplasia* 11, 1235-1242 (2009).

[37] Wu A C, He Y, Broomfield A, Paatan N J, Harrington B S, Tseng H W, Beaven E A, Kiernan D M, Swindle P, Clubb A B, Levesque J P, Winkler I G, Ling M T, Srinivasan B, Hooper J D, Pettit A R. CD169(+) macrophages mediate pathological

formation of woven bone in skeletal lesions of prostate cancer. *J. Pathol.* 239, 218-230 (2016).
[38] Movila A, Ishii T, Albassam A, Wisitrasameewong W, Howait M, Yamaguchi T, Ruiz-Torruella M, Bahammam L, Nishimura K, Van Dyke T, Kawai T. Macrophage Migration Inhibitory Factor (MIF) Supports Homing of Osteoclast Precursors to Peripheral Osteolytic Lesions. *J. Bone Miner. Res.* 31, 1688-1700 (2016).
[39] Cheng L, Ruan Z. Tim-3 and Tim-4 as the potential targets for antitumor therapy. *Hum. Vaccin. Immunother.* 11, 2458-2462 (2015).
[40] Roca H, Jones J D, Purica M C, Weidner S, Koh A J, Kuo R, Wilkinson J E, Wang Y, Daignault-Newton S, Pienta K J, Morgan T M, Keller E T, Nör J E, Shea L D, McCauley L K. Apoptosis-induced CXCL5 accelerates inflammation and growth of prostate tumor metastases in bone. *J. Clin. Invest.* 128, 248-266 (2018).
[41] Li X F, Selli C, Zhou H L, Cao J, Wu S, Ma R Y, Lu Y, Zhang C B, Xun B, Lam A D, Pang X C, Fernando A, Zhang Z, Unciti-Broceta A, Carragher N O, Ramachandran P, Henderson N C, Sun L L, Hu HY, Li G B, Sawyers C, Qian B Z. Macrophages promote anti-androgen resistance in prostate cancer bone disease. *J. Exp. Med.* 220, (2023).
[42] Batoon L, McCauley L K. Cross Talk Between Macrophages and Cancer Cells in the Bone Metastatic Environment. *Front Endocrinol. (Lausanne)* 12, 763846 (2021).
[43] Larson R C, Maus M V. Recent advances and discoveries in the mechanisms and functions of CAR T cells. *Nat. Rev. Cancer* 21, 145-161 (2021).
[44] Klichinsky M, Ruella M, Shestova O, Lu X M, Best A, Zeeman M, Schmierer M, Gabrusiewicz K, Anderson N R, Petty N E, Cummins K D, Shen F, Shan X, Veliz K, Blouch K, Yashiro-Ohtani Y, Kenderian SS, Kim M Y, O'Connor R S, Wallace S R, Kozlowski M S, Marchione D M, Shestov M, Garcia B A, June C H, Gill S. Human chimeric antigen receptor macrophages for cancer immunotherapy. *Nat. Biotechnol.* 38, 947-953 (2020).

Index

A

acid, 9, 15, 24, 29, 31, 55, 88, 97, 104, 106
adenocarcinoma, 33, 39, 98
adenosine, 3, 20, 78
adhesion, 14, 16, 25
algorithm, 45, 50, 52
alkaline phosphatase, viii, 41, 102, 104
angiogenesis, 28, 35, 36, 75, 107
antibody, 34, 36, 104
antigen, 28, 35, 36, 37, 73, 75, 107, 111
antitumor, 40, 79, 97, 111
apoptosis, 5, 10, 15, 25, 73, 105
asymptomatic, x, 42, 48, 86

B

back pain, viii, 41, 43, 66
base, 3, 22, 33
biomarkers, 18, 33, 37, 68, 79, 95, 108
biopsy, 33, 37, 39, 53, 55, 60, 64, 68
blood, viii, 33, 34, 41, 49, 54, 56, 64, 76, 87, 91, 105
body fluid, 28, 33, 34, 36
bone, vii, viii, ix, x, 1, 2, 3, 6, 8, 13, 14, 15, 16, 17, 18, 19, 23, 24, 25, 27, 28, 29, 30, 31, 32, 35, 36, 38, 39, 41, 42, 43, 44, 46, 47, 53, 54, 56, 57, 58, 63, 66, 68, 69, 71, 72, 73, 74, 75, 76, 77, 78, 79, 80, 81, 82, 83, 85, 86, 87, 88, 89, 90, 91, 92, 93, 94, 95, 96, 97, 98, 99, 100, 101, 102, 103, 104, 105, 106, 107, 108, 109, 110, 111
bone formation, 8, 29, 31, 54, 72, 101, 102, 104, 105, 106
bone homeostasis, ix, x, 2, 3, 71, 78, 82, 87, 88, 98, 99, 100, 101, 102, 105, 106, 107, 108
bone marrow, ix, x, 2, 29, 30, 32, 44, 71, 72, 73, 75, 76, 77, 82, 83, 85, 86, 87, 88, 89, 91, 92, 94, 95, 96, 98, 105, 110
bone matrix, viii, ix, x, 2, 6, 27, 29, 30, 71, 72, 75, 86, 87, 88, 93, 101
bone morphogenetic proteins (BMPs), viii, 27, 30, 88
bone remodeling, viii, 27, 30, 32, 33, 36, 76
bone resorption, viii, 27, 29, 30, 31, 43, 44, 72, 74, 75, 88, 93, 94, 95, 97, 101, 102, 103, 104, 106
bone scan, viii, 41, 54
breast cancer (BCa), vii, viii, ix, 2, 3, 16, 17, 26, 28, 30, 31, 35, 36, 38, 40, 47, 71, 72, 76, 77, 79, 81, 86, 89, 91, 92, 95, 96, 97, 98, 100, 101, 106, 110

C

calcium, viii, 32, 41, 86, 92
cancer, ii, vii, viii, ix, x, 1, 2, 3, 9, 13, 14, 15, 16, 17, 18, 19, 22, 24, 25, 26, 28, 29, 30, 31, 32, 33, 34, 35, 36, 37, 38, 39, 40, 42, 47, 68, 71, 72, 74, 76, 77, 78, 79, 80, 81, 82, 85, 86, 87, 88, 89, 91, 92, 93, 94, 95, 96, 97, 98, 99, 100, 101, 106, 107, 110, 111
cancer cells, ix, x, 14, 25, 31, 32, 35, 37, 38, 40, 72, 74, 76, 77, 85, 86, 87, 88, 89, 91, 92, 95, 96, 97, 98, 99, 106, 107, 110
cancer progression, vii, 1, 9, 35
candidates, 49, 56, 57

carcinoma, 25, 49, 54, 55, 82
CD8+, 73, 77, 82
cell differentiation, viii, 17, 27, 77
cell invasion, 10, 14, 15, 91
cell line, 9, 14, 31, 80
cerebrospinal fluid (CSF), viii, 27, 30, 47, 59, 74, 80, 102, 103, 104
chemotherapy, 8, 23, 43, 44, 48, 50, 51, 53, 60, 95
China, 1, 27, 71, 85, 99
classification, vii, 28, 49, 60, 61
clinical application, 33, 34, 35, 37, 101
coding, viii, 2, 4, 13, 17, 25, 28, 30
collagen, 14, 31, 38
colonization, ix, x, 71, 81, 86, 89, 91, 94, 95, 105
communication, 30, 36, 106
complications, vii, 1, 29, 56, 57, 58, 59
compression, viii, x, 2, 41, 42, 43, 44, 46, 47, 51, 52, 53, 54, 55, 57, 58, 59, 65, 66, 67, 69, 70, 86
compression fracture, viii, 41, 44, 46, 52, 54, 55, 58, 65
cortical bone, 54, 76, 104
CT scans, viii, 41, 42, 54
cure, 59, 60, 108
cytokines, viii, ix, x, 8, 10, 27, 43, 75, 76, 77, 80, 82, 85, 86, 87, 101, 102, 103, 104

D

death, ix, 24, 26, 46, 56, 82, 85, 86, 110
decay, 6, 10, 22, 26
deficiency, 73, 75, 77, 82
degradation, 3, 5, 7, 9, 10, 16
dendritic cell, 34, 35, 40, 73
deposition, 3, 38, 43
destruction, 42, 43, 46, 52, 53, 54, 91
detection, 34, 36, 42, 47, 54
diseases, 3, 6, 33, 36, 37, 46, 101, 108
disseminated tumor cells (DTC), x, 73, 86, 87, 89, 90, 91, 95, 97
distribution, 13, 17, 42, 43, 91
DNA, 2, 3, 13, 17, 18, 72

drugs, 13, 16, 17, 32, 33, 34, 36, 37, 55, 91

E

endothelial cells, 72, 76, 88, 91
environment, viii, 13, 28, 29, 32, 35, 53, 56, 71, 72, 73, 74, 75, 77, 78, 88, 92, 99
equilibrium, 7, 92, 101
erosion, ix, 53, 71, 102, 104
estrogen, v, vii, ix, 71, 72, 73, 74, 75, 76, 77, 78, 79, 80, 81, 82, 83
estrogen receptors, 71, 72, 78, 79
etiology, ii, vii, ix, 41
eukaryotic, 3, 6, 21, 23
evidence, vii, x, 1, 3, 4, 6, 33, 64, 67, 70, 73, 76, 99, 100, 101, 107
extracellular vesicles (EVs), vii, viii, 27, 28, 29, 30, 31, 32, 33, 34, 35, 36, 37, 38, 39

F

fibroblast growth factor (FGF), viii, 27, 30, 93
formation, ix, 6, 9, 10, 14, 15, 17, 23, 29, 31, 33, 72, 73, 76, 77, 81, 82, 86, 87, 88, 89, 93, 98, 101, 102, 103, 105, 106, 111
fractures, viii, x, 2, 29, 41, 44, 45, 46, 51, 52, 54, 55, 58, 65, 86, 100
fusion, 29, 31, 36, 52, 53

G

gene expression, 2, 3, 12, 23
genes, 4, 10, 12, 13, 102, 104
genetics, 19, 21, 22
genome, 8, 23, 72
glycolysis, 5, 10, 15, 20, 24
growth, viii, ix, x, 6, 8, 9, 10, 13, 15, 19, 23, 24, 27, 29, 30, 35, 36, 38, 43, 72, 73, 77, 81, 82, 85, 87, 88, 89, 92, 93, 94, 95, 97, 99, 101, 103, 104, 105, 106, 107, 110, 111
growth factor, viii, ix, 6, 27, 30, 35, 36, 43, 77, 82, 85, 87, 88, 89, 93, 95, 97, 103, 104

guidelines, 37, 46, 58, 68

H

health, viii, 41, 78, 82, 88
histology, 48, 51, 52
histone, 2, 3, 9, 13, 19
homeostasis, ix, x, 2, 3, 71, 78, 82, 87, 88, 98, 99, 100, 101, 102, 105, 106, 107, 108
hormones, ix, 72, 76, 85, 88, 93, 95, 96, 101, 109
human, 9, 10, 19, 20, 21, 28, 31, 35, 36, 38, 39, 55, 80, 81, 91, 95, 96, 97, 98, 108, 109
hypercalcemia, vii, 1, 2, 29, 44, 55

I

ideal, 17, 56, 58
identification, 5, 8, 17, 24
image, 47, 51, 53, 55, 56
immune response, 8, 28, 78, 100
immunological microenvironment, vii, ix, 71
immunotherapy, 22, 51, 100, 107, 111
in vitro, 13, 15, 104, 109
in vivo, 13, 15, 29, 76, 95, 97, 109
incidence, 22, 36, 42, 58, 65, 72, 73
induction, 13, 83, 94
inflammation, 43, 81, 111
inhibition, 16, 35, 80
inhibitor, 13, 35, 74, 94
initiation, 5, 6, 59
insulin, viii, 6, 27, 30, 93
insulin growth factor (IGF), viii, 27, 30, 93
integrin, 25, 35, 38, 43, 76, 82, 95, 96, 107
integrity, 4, 44, 88

K

kidney, viii, 34, 41, 42, 48

L

lead, 29, 32, 44, 46, 47, 49, 54, 73, 94, 103, 108
lesions, viii, ix, 2, 8, 27, 30, 31, 32, 41, 42, 44, 45, 47, 48, 52, 53, 54, 55, 58, 59, 60, 61, 62, 63, 64, 66, 68, 71, 88, 89, 93, 94, 95, 104, 106, 107, 111
life expectancy, 50, 52, 53, 57, 58, 59
ligand, 30, 43, 72, 73, 94, 103
liver, ix, 29, 37, 48, 49, 85, 86
liver cancer, ix, 29, 37, 48, 49, 85, 86
localization, 3, 4, 5
lung, viii, ix, 8, 14, 16, 17, 29, 30, 32, 36, 37, 39, 41, 42, 43, 44, 47, 48, 49, 54, 79, 85, 86, 89, 93, 98, 100
lung cancer (LCa), 14, 17, 30, 32, 37, 39, 42, 44, 47, 93, 100
lymphocytes, 28, 35, 37, 76
lymphoma, 47, 48, 51, 54, 58

M

macrophages, v, vii, x, 36, 73, 74, 75, 76, 79, 81, 82, 99, 100, 101, 102, 103, 104, 105, 106, 107, 108, 109, 110, 111
majority, 42, 46, 54, 55
malignant tumors, viii, ix, 27, 54, 71
management, vii, ix, 17, 22, 41, 42, 50, 51, 55, 66, 67, 68, 69
marrow, ix, x, 2, 29, 30, 32, 42, 44, 54, 71, 72, 73, 75, 76, 77, 82, 83, 85, 86, 87, 88, 89, 91, 92, 94, 95, 96, 98, 105, 110
mass, 4, 30, 54, 72, 100
matrix, viii, ix, x, 2, 6, 27, 28, 29, 30, 31, 71, 72, 75, 77, 86, 87, 88, 93, 95, 101
matrix metallopeptidase (MMP), 14, 16, 25, 31
medical, 25, 50, 51, 52, 53, 60, 100
men, 31, 78, 86
mesenchymal stem cells, 32, 82, 87, 95, 103, 108, 110
messenger RNA (mRNA), 2, 3, 4, 5, 6, 9, 10, 13, 14, 17, 19, 20, 21, 22, 23, 24, 25, 26, 33, 39

Index

metabolism, vii, ix, 1, 6, 7, 16, 20, 71, 72, 75, 86, 92

metastasis, vii, viii, ix, x, 1, 2, 3, 6, 8, 9, 13, 14, 15, 16, 17, 18, 25, 26, 27, 28, 29, 30, 31, 32, 33, 35, 36, 37, 38, 39, 40, 41, 42, 43, 46, 49, 52, 54, 57, 58, 59, 65, 66, 67, 68, 69, 71, 72, 73, 74, 75, 77, 78, 79, 80, 81, 82, 83, 85, 86, 87, 88, 89, 90, 91, 92, 93, 94, 95, 96, 97, 98, 99, 100, 101, 103, 104, 105, 106, 107, 108, 110

metastatic disease, 41, 42, 44, 46, 53, 54, 65, 66, 67, 68, 91

methylation, 3, 5, 6, 8, 9, 14, 15, 17, 19, 20, 21, 24

methyltransferase complex (MTC), 3, 4, 7

mice, 5, 73, 77, 82, 83, 97

migration, 9, 10, 14, 15, 23, 24, 28, 36, 83, 106

mineralization, 29, 31, 101

modifications, 2, 3, 4, 6, 9, 13, 14, 19

molecules, 18, 28, 35, 36, 37, 92

morbidity, 2, 56, 64

mortality, vii, x, 1, 2, 36, 56, 87, 99, 100

motif, 4, 5, 10, 103

multiple myeloma, viii, 28, 34, 47, 54, 56, 58

N

N(6)-methyladenosine (m6A), vii, 1, 2, 21, 22, 24

necrosis, 9, 56, 77, 103

nerve, 42, 44, 55, 59, 63

neurologic, oncologic, mechanical instability, and systemic disease (NOMS), 50, 52, 67

non-coding RNAs (lncRNAs), 4, 13, 17

nucleus, 5, 6, 72, 109

O

opportunities, 23, 66, 97

organs, ix, 16, 29, 32, 35, 58, 72, 85, 86, 87, 88, 89, 95, 97, 110

osteoblasts, viii, ix, x, 17, 27, 28, 29, 30, 31, 38, 72, 73, 74, 75, 76, 85, 86, 87, 88, 89, 92, 93, 94, 97, 98, 99, 101, 102, 103, 104, 105, 109

osteoclastogenesis, viii, x, 27, 31, 32, 38, 39, 79, 80, 86, 89, 98, 109

osteoclasts, viii, ix, x, 8, 17, 27, 28, 29, 30, 33, 43, 72, 73, 74, 75, 76, 77, 79, 80, 82, 85, 86, 87, 93, 99, 101, 102, 103, 104, 105, 106, 109

osteolytic, viii, ix, x, 8, 16, 17, 23, 26, 27, 30, 31, 32, 41, 53, 54, 68, 71, 73, 86, 89, 93, 96, 104, 106, 107, 111

osteosarcoma (OS), vii, viii, 2, 3, 6, 8, 9, 10, 12, 13, 15, 22, 23, 24, 25, 28, 80

osteosclerotic, viii, 41, 54, 68

P

pain, vii, viii, 1, 2, 33, 41, 43, 44, 45, 51, 52, 55, 56, 57, 58, 59, 60, 64, 66, 68, 82, 100

paralysis, 47, 48, 58, 67

parathyroid hormone, 76, 93, 95, 96, 109

pathogenesis, vii, ix, 12, 41, 79, 96, 98

pathway, 8, 9, 10, 12, 13, 14, 16, 18, 24, 25, 33, 36, 37, 39, 72, 78, 80, 87, 92, 94, 96, 98, 100, 103, 107, 108, 109

PET scans, viii, 41, 54

phenotype, 17, 26, 38, 73, 100, 101, 103, 106

phosphate, 10, 30, 86

phosphorylation, 14, 16, 72

plasticity, 95, 100, 101, 104, 107

platelet-derived growth factor (PDGF), viii, 27, 30, 35

platform, 36, 39, 51

plexus, viii, 41, 43, 65

polarization, 75, 81, 100, 106

population, 22, 83, 103

prevention, 52, 93, 105

primary tumor, ix, 2, 30, 42, 47, 56, 60, 85, 87, 88, 89, 91, 105, 107

progenitor cells, 29, 33, 73, 87

prognosis, 8, 9, 14, 16, 17, 18, 25, 33, 34, 37, 44, 48, 52, 87

pro-inflammatory, 74, 75, 103

Index

proliferation, vii, viii, 1, 9, 10, 13, 14, 15, 23, 24, 25, 28, 30, 31, 35, 38, 82, 88, 91, 93, 94, 102, 104, 106
promoter, 9, 14, 77
prostate cancer (PCa), vii, ix, 1, 2, 3, 13, 14, 16, 17, 25, 31, 38, 42, 48, 71, 72, 74, 76, 78, 81, 86, 88, 91, 92, 95, 96, 97, 100, 101, 106, 107, 110, 111
protein, viii, 3, 4, 5, 6, 7, 9, 10, 12, 13, 14, 17, 18, 21, 22, 23, 28, 30, 31, 32, 33, 34, 35, 36, 37, 49, 76, 88, 93, 95, 96, 104

R

radiation, 44, 46, 48, 50, 51, 52, 57, 58, 59, 60, 69
radioresistant, viii, 41, 46, 49, 51, 57, 58, 59, 68
radiosensitive, viii, 41, 48, 50, 51, 55, 58, 68
radiotherapy, viii, 41, 43, 46, 48, 50, 51, 53, 54, 57, 58, 59, 63, 65, 68, 69
receptor, ix, 9, 30, 34, 35, 36, 71, 72, 73, 78, 79, 89, 93, 94, 97, 103, 107, 111
receptor activator of nuclear factor kappa-B ligand (RANKL), viii, x, 16, 27, 30, 32, 39, 73, 77, 81, 86, 93, 102, 103, 104, 109
recognition, 5, 13, 14, 21, 23
reconstruction, 29, 53, 63
recurrence, 8, 60, 63, 94
regeneration, viii, ix, 27, 71
relevance, 34, 37, 97
relief, 45, 51, 55, 56, 57, 58, 60, 64
renal cell carcinoma, 48, 49, 59
repair, ix, 13, 29, 86, 109
resection, 34, 36, 60, 62, 63, 70
resistance, 9, 15, 16, 24, 32, 107, 111
response, 8, 20, 29, 48, 51, 57, 74, 75, 81, 88, 93, 95, 100, 105, 106
risk, 44, 45, 46, 59, 73, 94
RNA, vii, viii, 1, 2, 3, 4, 5, 6, 7, 9, 10, 12, 13, 14, 15, 16, 17, 18, 19, 20, 21, 22, 23, 24, 25, 26, 28, 30, 31, 33, 34, 38, 39, 81
RNA splicing, vii, 1, 3, 7

roots, 42, 44, 59, 63

S

safety, 17, 48, 69
secrete, x, 29, 35, 37, 38, 86, 88, 89, 102, 103, 104, 106
secretion, 29, 31, 35, 37, 88, 95, 101, 107
seeding, 42, 89, 91
separation surgery, 41, 50, 63, 64, 70
serum, viii, 34, 41
sex, 4, 19, 73
shape, 8, 56, 92
signaling pathway, 9, 12, 13, 14, 16, 18, 24, 25, 72, 92, 103, 107
signalling, 78, 80, 94
signals, 2, 28, 73, 87, 88, 89, 93
skeletal-related events (SREs), 29, 32, 44, 55, 66
skeleton, 29, 80, 88, 92
solid tumors, vii, ix, 1, 36, 65, 71, 86
spinal cord, 42, 44, 47, 48, 51, 57, 58, 59, 63, 64, 65, 66, 67, 69, 70
spinal metastasis, vii, ix, 41, 42, 54, 57, 58, 59, 65, 67, 68, 69
spine, v, viii, 41, 42, 44, 45, 46, 47, 49, 50, 52, 53, 54, 56, 57, 58, 59, 63, 64, 65, 66, 67, 68, 69, 70
spread, viii, ix, 33, 41, 42, 43, 60, 85, 86, 91
stability, vii, viii, 1, 4, 5, 6, 9, 10, 13, 14, 15, 16, 21, 22, 24, 25, 41, 46, 51, 54, 55, 56, 67, 77
stabilization, 20, 25, 44, 45, 46, 50, 51, 52, 60, 64, 66
stem cells, 8, 23, 32, 82, 87, 91, 92, 95, 96, 103, 108, 110
stereotactic body radiotherapy (SBRT), 41, 50, 58, 63, 68, 69
steroids, 43, 55, 73
stimulation, 31, 38, 43, 55, 68, 81, 89
stroma, 22, 29, 89, 110
stromal cells, x, 8, 76, 77, 87, 99
structure, 3, 4, 6
substrate, 3, 4, 6, 20, 21, 88

Index

surgery, viii, 8, 41, 49, 50, 51, 52, 56, 57, 58, 59, 60, 63, 64, 69, 70, 85, 100, 108
survival, 2, 8, 10, 15, 22, 43, 46, 48, 49, 51, 52, 57, 63, 66, 73, 87, 92, 94, 107
survival rate, 8, 10, 22
symptoms, x, 99, 100
synthesis, 5, 13, 29

T

T cells, 28, 32, 73, 76, 77, 79, 81, 82, 83, 107, 111
target, 4, 5, 6, 10, 13, 15, 16, 17, 35, 43, 58, 87, 89, 91, 106, 107
techniques, 51, 56, 64, 65, 108
therapeutic targets, x, 18, 35, 37, 86, 93, 94, 106
therapy, 2, 8, 16, 17, 24, 25, 33, 34, 36, 37, 39, 51, 55, 56, 58, 59, 65, 77, 82, 100, 101, 107, 111
thyroid, viii, 41, 42, 43, 48, 49, 55
tissue, viii, ix, 8, 9, 14, 28, 33, 34, 37, 43, 46, 54, 56, 71, 85, 86, 100, 101, 103, 108, 109
TNF, 75, 102, 103, 105, 109
TNF-α, 75, 102, 103, 105
transcription, 9, 14, 16, 23, 32, 35, 72, 80, 91, 98
transcripts, 5, 6, 8, 17
transforming growth factor (TGF), viii, 27, 30, 77, 82, 91, 93, 102, 104
transforming growth factor beta (TGF-β), viii, 27, 30, 91, 102, 104
translation, vii, 1, 3, 5, 6, 7, 9, 10, 15, 16, 19, 22, 26, 45
translocation, 3, 32, 109
treatment, vii, viii, x, 1, 2, 3, 8, 13, 17, 23, 28, 29, 33, 34, 36, 41, 42, 45, 46, 47, 48, 49, 50, 51, 52, 53, 55, 57, 58, 59, 60, 63, 64, 67, 68, 69, 78, 86, 91, 93, 94, 99, 100, 101, 104, 105, 106, 107, 108
triggers, 35, 40, 97
tropism, 29, 31, 89
tumor associated macrophages (TAMs), 100, 106, 107
tumor cells, ix, x, 2, 14, 16, 29, 30, 32, 35, 36, 38, 43, 73, 83, 85, 86, 87, 88, 89, 90, 91, 92, 93, 94, 95, 96, 97, 105, 106, 107
tumor growth, x, 10, 13, 15, 35, 77, 97, 99, 101, 106, 107, 110
tumor invasion, 60, 75, 100
tumor metastasis, 28, 82, 89, 100, 107
tumor necrosis factor, 9, 77, 103
tumor progression, 24, 25, 35, 76
tumorigenesis, vii, 1, 9, 24, 33
tumors, vii, viii, ix, x, 1, 2, 3, 6, 8, 9, 10, 12, 13, 14, 15, 16, 17, 23, 24, 25, 27, 28, 29, 30, 32, 33, 34, 35, 36, 37, 38, 39, 40, 41, 42, 43, 44, 45, 46, 47, 48, 49, 51, 52, 53, 54, 55, 56, 57, 58, 59, 60, 63, 65, 66, 67, 69, 70, 71, 74, 75, 76, 77, 78, 81, 82, 83, 85, 86, 87, 88, 89, 91, 92, 93, 94, 96, 97, 98, 99, 100, 103, 105, 106, 107, 108, 110, 111

U

underlying mechanisms, 18, 104, 105
United States, 21, 22, 82

V

vascular endothelial growth factor (VEGF), 74, 75, 88, 89
vertebrae, 13, 42, 43, 44, 46, 59, 60, 61, 65, 66
vesicle, 28, 38, 39, 40
vicious cycle, x, 8, 86, 92, 93, 97

W

Wnt signaling, 8, 13, 25
women, 44, 73, 78, 79, 86
worldwide, ix, 2, 13, 85, 86, 107